THE INFLUENCES OF PANCREATIC TUMORS ON THE STOMACH

To John I. Hollenbeck
from one author
to another!
[illegible] M. Tollinger
Mar. 1974.

THE INFLUENCES OF PANCREATIC TUMORS ON THE STOMACH

By

ROBERT M. ZOLLINGER, M.D., F.A.C.S.

Regents Professor and Chairman
Department of Surgery
The Ohio State University College of Medicine
Columbus, Ohio

and

DAVID W. COLEMAN

Administrative Assistant and Program Director
Islet Cell Tumor Studies
Department of Surgery
The Ohio State University College of Medicine
Columbus, Ohio

With a Foreword by

R.A. Gregory, C.BE., F.R.S.

The George Holt Professor of Physiology
University of Liverpool
Liverpool, England

CHARLES C THOMAS • PUBLISHER

Springfield • Illinois • U.S.A.

Published and Distributed Throughout the World by
CHARLES C THOMAS • PUBLISHER
BANNERSTONE HOUSE
301-327 East Lawrence Avenue, Springfield, Illinois, U.S.A.

ISBN 0-398-02683-1
Library of Congress Catalog Card Number: 72-88460

Printed in the United States of America

EE-11

FIFTIETH ANNUAL BEAUMONT LECTURE

Wayne County Medical Society

Detroit, Michigan

Dedicated to

EDWIN H. ELLISON, M.D.

Professor of Surgery
Ohio State University
Columbus, Ohio
1957-1958

Professor of Surgery and Chairman of the Division of Surgery
Marquette University
Milwaukee, Wisconsin
1958-1970

With gratitude for his many contributions to the ulcerogenic islet cell syndrome.

FOREWORD

It is not only a privilege but also a great personal pleasure for me to introduce this book.

For years now, Robert Zollinger's many friends and admirers have been urging him to write this account of what is recognized to be one of the most significant discoveries of recent years in regard to the problem of peptic ulceration and the implication therein of the antral hormone gastrin. Zollinger and Ellison were not the first to observe that in certain cases of severe and intractable duodenal ulceration there was to be found a tumour of the pancreas; but they were the first to perceive the element of causality in this relationship and to suggest that it was the excessive and unrestrained production by the pancreatic tumour of a potent gastric secretagogue, resulting in profound hypersecretion of gastric acid, which was the basis of the dramatic and often catastrophic clinical picture. Subsequent studies have completely confirmed their original hypothesis; it has been established that in such cases, the pancreatic tumour elaborates and secretes into the circulation hormones which are identical with those which have been extracted from human antral mucosa and are normally responsible for an important phase in the postprandial stimulation of gastric acid secretion. As will be clear to readers of this monograph, there is a large and rapidly growing field of study of what the author modestly prefers to term the "ulcerogenic syndrome," involving not only the surgeon but also the histologist, the pathologist, and the biochemist. The introduction of radioimmunoassay for plasma gastrin is showing that the condition, particularly in a relatively mild form, is much more common than was originally supposed. There is a still-obscure relationship to the syndrome of multiple endocrine adenomatosis and to the equally remarkable condition of "pancreatic cholera" which is likewise associated with a pancreatic tumour. Differentiation of the islet cell types in the pancreas and alignment of them with the cellular components of tumours of that organ presents a challenging problem for the histologist. The biochemist is not only concerned with isolation and identification of the hormonal principles but will also see in the ZE tumour a unique possibility of studying in surviving tissue slices or perhaps cultured cells the cellular mechanisms of hormonal biosynthesis. It is safe to prophesy that this multidisciplinary study of the Zollinger-Ellison syndrome will bring a rich harvest of new information bearing not only upon the clinical basis of peptic ulceration but also upon the fundamental biology of the gastrointestinal hormone-secreting cells.

Dr. Zollinger's unique relationship to his subject and the definitive review he presents of its many problems must make this book compulsory reading for everyone interested in the gastrointestinal tract. Not only "compulsory" but also "compulsive" reading; for it is a fascinating story, and no one is better fitted to tell it than he who, with the late Edwin Ellison, started it all.

R. A. Gregory

PREFACE

MAN VS. MURIATIC ACID

Since the beginning of time, man has been concerned with providing sufficient food to control his hunger pains. He had shown little concern for how the stomach meets the daily challenge of his dietary irregularities until William Beaumont's observations, between 1823 and 1833, on the role of muriatic or hydrochloric acid and various foods on the process of digestion.

Beaumont's observations on Alexis St. Martin clearly defined the phenomena which occurred in the stomach during digestion, the precise mode of action and the nature of the juice, its action inside as well as outside the body, and the influence of intemperance and unwholesome diet on digestion. His studies on the digestibility of various foods in the stomach are said to be the most important contributions ever made to practical dietetics. Likewise, the idea of applying surgical methods to investigations of the gastrointestinal tract was inspired by the gunshot wound which had left St. Martin with the hole in his stomach. Since that time, thousands of experiments and observations have been made every year in an effort to clarify the many unresolved mysteries of digestion (Fig. 1).

MAN vs. "MURIATIC ACID"
Gastric HCl identified 1824-1833
Influenced by: Temperature, Foods, etc. (Beaumont)
"Conditioned reflexes" (Pavlov)
Gastrin and secretin
Vagotomy, antrectomy
Islet cell tumors
Diagnosis by immunoassay

Figure 1. Since the time of Beaumont, the mechanisms involved in the production and control of gastric acidity have been a constant interest to both research investigators and clinicians.

This monograph was developed from a presentation made on the Fiftieth Annual Beaumont Lecture before the Wayne County Medical Society of Detroit. It is primarily concerned with the role of certain non-beta islet cell tumors of the pancreas and their influences on the stomach and its production of hydrochloric acid. These tumors have proven to be a potent extragastric source of both hormonal stimulation and inhibition of gastric acid secretion, and they are associated with recognizable, often life-threatening, clinical syndromes.

A digest of the available material concerning the "ulcerogenic" and "diarrheogenic" islet cell tumor syndromes will be presented, together with a commentary on the life and contributions of William Beaumont, whom Dragstedt recently named America's

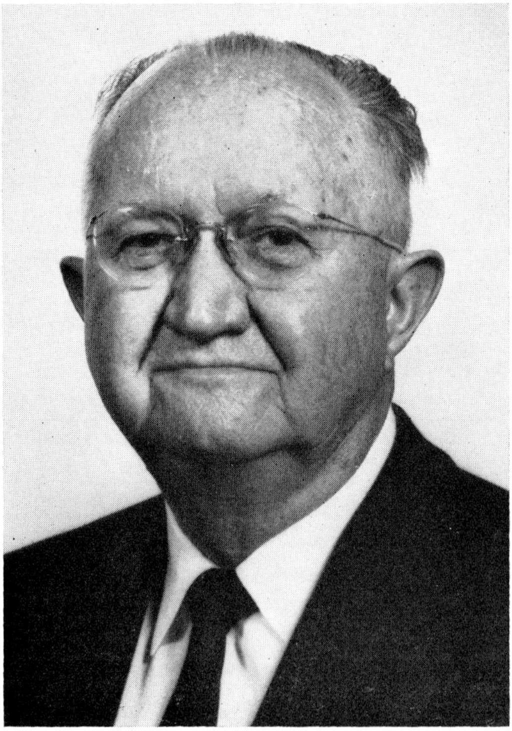

Figure 2. Dr. Lester R. Dragstedt, distinguished gastrointestinal physiologist and surgeon.

first Surgeon-Scientist (Fig. 2). On the fiftieth anniversary of this Society, it would also seem appropriate that attention be directed to the fact that there remains a tremendous challenge to all of us in helping man to combat his tendency to make too much or too little hydrochloric acid.

ACKNOWLEDGMENT

This work was supported by a grant from The John A. Hartford Foundation, Inc., New York, New York; National Institute of General Medical Sciences Grant GM-1539-06; and United States Public Health Service Grant RR-34.

CONTENTS

THE INFLUENCES OF PANCREATIC TUMORS ON THE STOMACH

Section I

DEVELOPMENT OF THE ULCEROGENIC ISLET CELL TUMOR CONCEPT

DR. ERNEST HENRY STARLING, in the first of his Croonian Lectures to the Royal College of Physicians of London on June 20, 1905, first used the word hormone to describe the action of an extract of duodenum, designated secretin, which he and his brother-in-law, Sir William Maddock Bayliss, had discovered three years earlier.[715,717] Starling also used the term in his third lecture to define the action of gastrin ("gastric secretin") which had been extracted from the gastric antrum by J. S. Edkins and reported to the Royal Society of London on May 18, 1905.[719] He said that both secretin and gastrin met the requirements of a hormone, or chemical messenger:

> These chemical messengers, however, or "hormones" (from ὁρμάω I excite or arouse), as we might call them, have to be carried from the organ where they are produced to the organ which they affect by means of the blood stream and the continually recurring physiological needs of the organism must determine their repeated production and circulation through the body.

For another half century or more, it was not apparent to either physiologists or clinicians that these chemical messengers could be produced outside the stomach or duodenum or that they might be elaborated in excessive amounts by certain endocrine tumors of the pancreas. Further, it was not appreciated that excesses of either hormone could cause a recognizable clinical syndrome. The implication of the first two gastrointestinal hormones, secretin and gastrin, in distinct clinical syndromes caused by non-beta islet cell tumors of the pancreas is the subject of this story.

A direct relationship between non–insulin–producing islet cell tumors and a pancreatic phase of gastric hypersecretion was first advanced on April 29, 1955, at the annual meeting in Philadelphia of the American Surgical Association. The paper was entitled: "Primary Peptic Ulcerations of the Jejunum Associated with Islet Cell Tumors of the Pancreas."[1] At that time, an ulcerogenic humoral factor of pancreatic islet origin was postulated and a diagnostic triad for a new clinical syndrome proposed, consisting of:

1. The presence of primary ulcerations in unusual locations, i.e. second or third portions of the duodenum, upper jejunum, or recurrent stomal ulcers following any type of gastric surgery short of total gastrectomy.
2. Gastric hypersecretion of gigantic proportions persisting despite adequate conventional medical, surgical or irradiation therapy.
3. The identification of non-specific islet cell tumors of the pancreas (Fig. 3).

This triad was suggested as a result of the very trying clinical experiences with two patients starting in early 1952. Both had primary jejunal ulcerations with stubborn ulcer recurrences, despite all of the traditionally accepted forms of medical and surgical treatment, short of total gastrectomy.

Both patients were women, one 36 and the other 19 years of age. So severe and catastrophic were their ulcer symptoms that Dr. Ellison and I sought consultation as well as consolation with

DIAGNOSTIC TRIAD

1. **Fulminating ulcer diathesis (12-hr secretion, 2-3 liters).**
2. **Rapidly recurring ulceration despite adequate therapy:**
   - **a. medical**
   - **b. surgical**
   - **c. radiation**
3. **Non-beta islet cell tumor of the pancreas.**

Figure 3. The original diagnostic triad proposed in 1955 describes the basic requirements for the diagnosis of an ulcerogenic islet cell tumor of the pancreas.

each other at frequent intervals during 1954. Every surgical clinic has had the experience of being unable to explain a few surgical failures with recurrent ulcerations despite the fact that one or more traditional operations for ulcer had been carried out with expertise.

The older patient, in the initial report, was first seen by the late Dr. Edwin H. Ellison on referral from Dr. Harry Burley of Springfield, Ohio, and Dr. Richard Fulton of Columbus, Ohio, in July, 1952. Within 30 days, because of recurrent massive hemorrhage, she underwent two sleeve resections of the upper jejunum for an ulcer just beyond the ligament of Treitz. She had had no previous upper gastrointestinal surgery. The patient continued to have massive upper gastrointestinal hemorrhages and a recurrent jejunal ulcer, despite a subsequent transabdominal vagotomy and two gastric resections (Fig. 4). It is very doubtful that the significance of the acid factor was truly appreciated in the early surgical management of this patient, but the shattering effect caused by the prompt recurrence of hemorrhages was not forgotten by the surgeon. A vivid picture of the problem, which Sircus has recently described as "an intractable saga of peptic ulceration,"[606] can be appreciated from Dr. Ellison's description of the patient's final year of life. She was observed between July, 1952, and the time of her demise in June 1954, a period of almost three years.

> At the time of an elective admission in January, 1953, for reevaluation, the patient weighed 105 pounds and was symptom-free. The twelve-hour overnight gastric aspiration yielded 1,005 ml, with 29 mEq of free hydrochloric acid. Barium studies were negative. The patient was discharged without medication and continued to improve for the next month. However, the severe epigastric pain recurred and resulted in her fourth hospital admission on July 29, 1953. The twelve-hour secretion approximated 800 ml with 26.4 mEq of free hydrochloric acid. She had lost twelve pounds in weight since January, 1953, and a marked deficit in blood volume was noted. A course of intensive ulcer therapy was instituted and the patient was discharged to her family physician.
>
> The symptoms were controlled with therapy previously advised until October, 1953, at which time a marginal ulceration was demon-

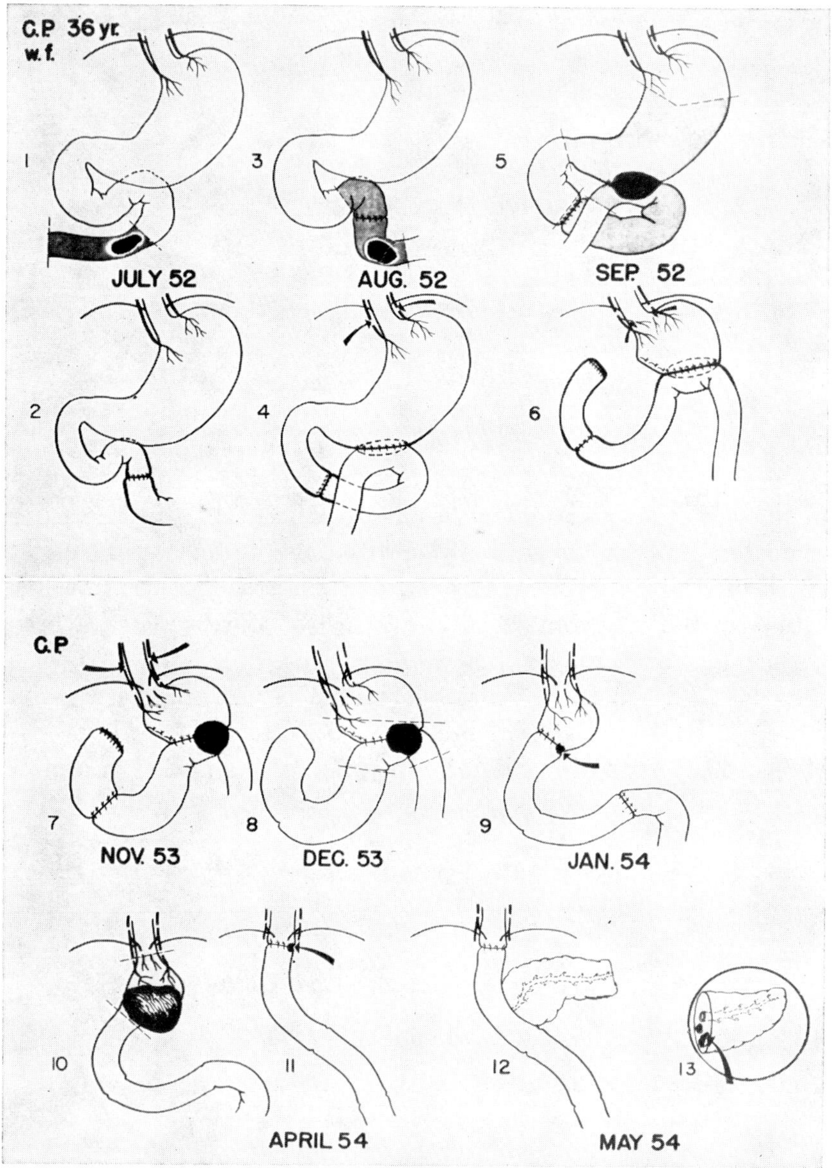

Figure 4. Schematic drawings to illustrate the six operations carried out on one of the two patients in the original report of the ulcerogenic syndrome.

strated by roentgenogram. In November, 1953, she was admitted to her local hospital where a transthoracic vagotomy had failed to control her progressive symptoms or alter a positive Hollander test. The milliequivalents of free hydrochloric acid exceeded 100 at the time that the twelve-hour overnight secretion studies were made. One month later, the marginal ulcer was excised, the additional stomach was removed, and continuity restored by gastroduodenostomy. The postoperative course was stormy, and following an episode of chills and fever, a gastroenterocutaneous fistula appeared which drained various amounts of gastrointestinal secretions that made electrolyte maintenance a difficult problem.

When transferred to University Hospital [fifth admission] in February, 1954, her weight had fallen to 72 pounds. It was obvious that the patient's ability to produce larger volumes of gastric juice rich in hydrochloric acid was slowly but surely increasing, regardless of two vagotomies and numerous other gastric procedures. The patient's general condition improved but the gastric fistula remained unchanged and accordingly was approached surgically on April 2, 1954. The gastroduodenostomy appeared to have separated completely, except for one small area on the lesser curvature side. The open duodenum and gastric pouch communicated with a large, thick-walled cavity which completely surrounded the lower end of the stomach. Any definite procedure was considered out of the question. A large Pezzar catheter was inserted in the gastric pouch and was brought to the outside in an attempt to divert the acid gastric juice away from the ulcerated area. A smaller but longer catheter was placed in the open end of the duodenum for feeding purposes, and the cavity itself was packed with gauze. Prior to closure, a large walled-off abscess in the right lower quadrant was drained to the outside.

Drainage from the gastric pouch varied from 1,625 ml to 4,750 ml and averaged 3,750 ml in spite of the patient's taking nothing by mouth. Free hydrochloric acid was present in the amount of 56 mEq/L and averaged 106 mEq during each twelve-hour period. The free hydrochloric acid was neutralized with sodium bicarbonate and all of the collected secretions were then returned to the gastrointestinal tract by means of the duodenostomy. Two weeks later the patient suffered two successive massive gastrointestinal hemorrhages, requiring 18 pints of whole blood to replace the loss. Continued bleeding necessitated total gastrectomy with esophagoduodenostomy which was accomplished on April 14, 1954.

> A duodenoesophagocutaneous fistula, from which large amounts of bile and jejunal contents were draining, gradually led to her demise on June 7, 1954.

It is significant that at the time of postmortem examination, gross examination of the pancreas did not reveal evidence of a tumor; however, there was a notation of hypertrophy and hyperplasia of the adrenal glands. No mention was made of an adenoma of the pancreas in the gross anatomical description; but subsequent microscopic examination did show several nodules of various sizes. The larger ones, measuring almost 1 cm in diameter, were found in the central portion of the pancreas. There were several other nodules present, some of which were hardly greater in size than an islet. It was concluded at that time that the pancreatic nodules were islet cell tumors of undetermined type which did not contain beta cells.

The second patient, a 19-year-old single girl, was admitted to the Emergency Room of University Hospital on January 19, 1954, on referral from Dr. C. C. Landen of Columbus, Ohio. A tentative diagnosis of intestinal obstruction was made because of the severe vomiting and abdominal pain of 14 hours' duration. The patient had had a rather complicated clinical and surgical history starting in July, 1951, when she was only 16 years of age. Her appendix was removed in 1952, and in July, 1953, after a bout of severe, acute abdominal pain, celiotomy was performed, at which time two separate perforated jejunal ulcers, located six inches from the ligament of Treitz, were identified and closed primarily.

During the interval from July, 1951, until November, 1953, the patient had lost 59 pounds from her original weight of 180. X-ray studies were made because of the suspicion of intestinal obstruction, and Miller-Abbott intubation was instituted. Barium by mouth showed slight dilatation of the small intestine with segmentation, but no obstruction. The barium was noted in the cecum within 45 minutes, and there were no jejunal ulcerations seen. Four days after admission, a 12-hour gastric aspiration produced a volume of 2,800 ml with 300 mEq of free acid. The next day, 2,400 ml of gastric aspiration contained 259 mEq of free hydrochloric acid. The fasting blood sugar level was 102 mg%.

A repeat upper gastrointestinal series showed considerable hypersecretion, a possible duodenal ulcer in the apical portion of the duodenal bulb, and a sacculation behind the stomach suggestive of upper jejunal ulceration. The small bowel again was noted to present a picture of coarseness and segmentation.

Because of the gigantic amounts of hydrochloric acid being produced by the patient and because she was less than 20 years of age, it was decided that a conservative type of operation was indicated; but at the same time, an heroic effort would be made to control the marked gastric hypersecretion. Accordingly, on January 28, 1954, subdiaphragmatic vagotomy, radical gastrectomy with fundusectomy and end-to-end gastroduodenostomy were accomplished (Fig. 5). The residual gastric pouch measured only 6 cm by 8 cm. The fundus of the stomach had been removed in an effort to cut down the amount of gastric secretion, a procedure recommended in 1931 by F. G. Connell of Oshkosh, Wisconsin.[723]

A colored motion picture was taken of the operation because of the technical approach being utilized to control the marked gastric hypersecretion in such a young patient. It was planned to submit this motion picture for review by the Motion Picture Committee of the American College of Surgeons for possible inclusion in the following year's Clinical Congress.

Within 10 days after the operation, however, the patient began to develop precordial burning and midline pain requiring narcotics for control. The gastric aspiration again showed a 12-hour volume of 570 ml with 28 mEq of free hydrochloric acid. Within 24 hours after discharge from the hospital on February 14, 1954, she was readmitted because of severe cramping and right upper quadrant pain. She had vomited twice and the vomitus in one instance was bloody. She responded temporarily to intensive antacid therapy but had to be readmitted within four and one-half months, on July 14, 1954. The patient had followed her diet religiously, gaining weight up to 147 pounds. While receiving a vagal blocking agent, a repeat 12-hour gastric aspiration showed 2,000 ml of gastric juice with a total of 32 mEq of free acid, despite the fact that she had undergone vagotomy and possessed

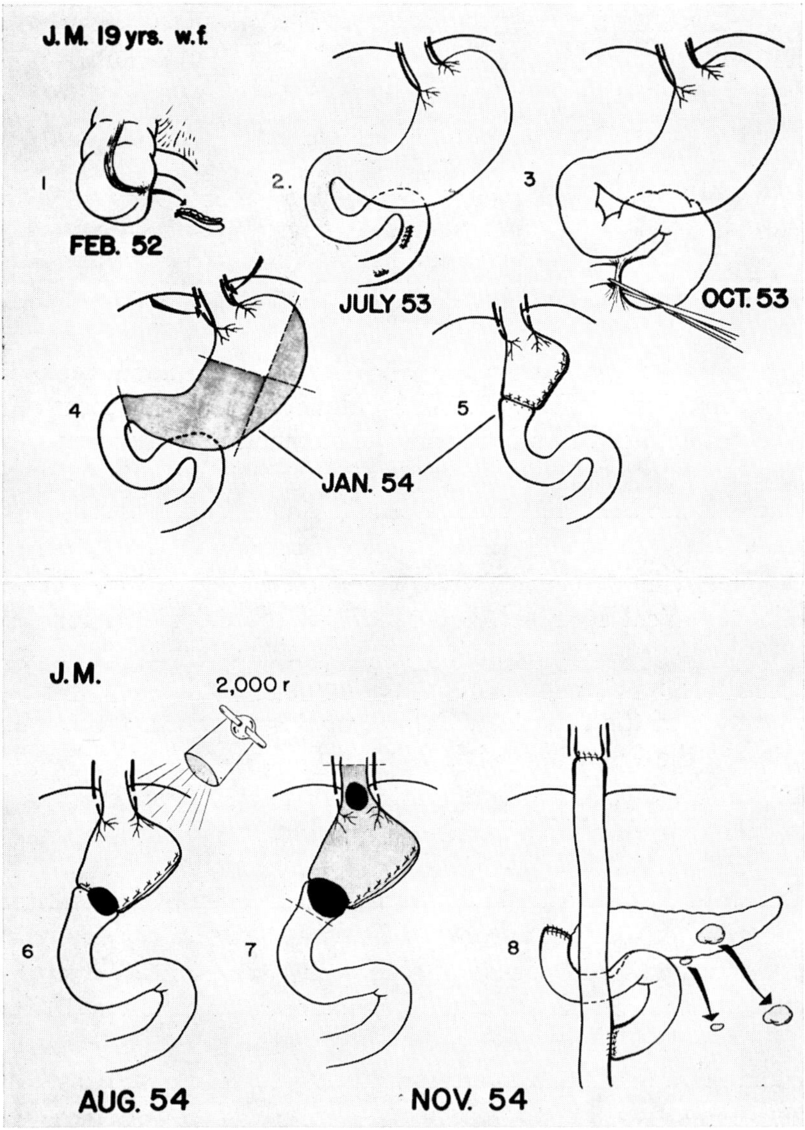

Figure 5. The diagrammatic outline of the various surgical and roentgenological treatment carried out in one of the two initial reported cases. Islet cell tumor was found on the surface of the pancreas, with metastases in an adjacent lymph node at the time of total gastrectomy.[1]

a gastric remnant only 6 by 8 cm in size. Roentgenologic studies, repeated in July, 1954, demonstrated a herniation of the fundus through an enlarged hiatal opening. There also appeared to be a small barium pocket, projecting on the greater curvature side, suggesting the possibility of an ulcer crater.

Still unwilling to accept the inevitability of total gastrectomy in so young a patient, it was decided to try roentgen therapy in the hope of bringing the acid factor under control. A total of 100 roentgen units twice weekly were directed to the area of the gastric pouch, until July 24, 1954, when a dosage of 2,000 had

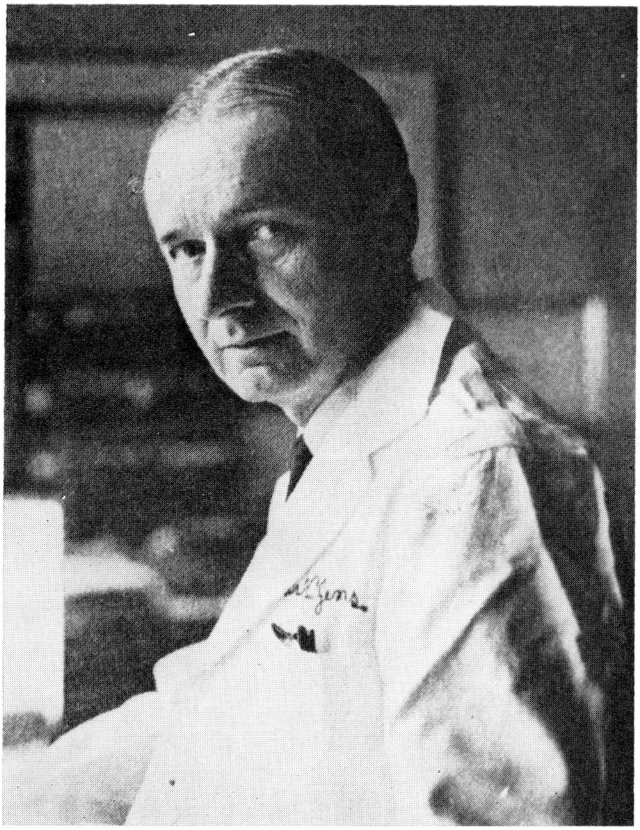

Figure 6. A photograph of Dr. Hilger Jenkins of the Department of Surgery, University of Chicago, who suggested that a tumor of the pancreas should be considered at the time of reoperation in Case 2.

been achieved (Fig. 5). The excruciating, burning epigastric pain continued and proved to be unresponsive to medication, necessitating continuous aspiration of the gastric contents for periods of 48 hours. In spite of the roentgen therapy, gastric aspiration showed an overnight volume of 1,350 ml with a total of 81.9 mEq of free acid—all from a gastric pouch no bigger than an orange.

We had written to Dr. Hilger P. Jenkins, then Chairman of the Motion Picture Committee of the American College of Surgeons (Figure 6), indicating that our "dream operation" for the control of marked gastric hypersecretion had failed, and that obviously, the motion picture made at the time of fundusectomy, vagotomy, and gastroduodenostomy should not be shown. On August 5, 1954, Dr. Jenkins replied:

> This reminds me a bit of a case that I had of multiple gastric, duodenal and jejunal ulcerations, and ultimate perforation in a lady that had an islet cell tumor of the pancreas. She was apparently carrying out a constant insulin test on her gastroduodenal-jejunal mechanism, which was her undoing. Is there any possibility that your little girl has a touch of hyperinsulinism as an etiology for this interesting condition (Fig. 7).

Certainly, Dr. Jenkins should be given full credit for suggesting that an islet cell tumor of the pancreas be thoroughly considered at the time of reexploration. It was for this reason that the patient was fasted for 48 hours with repeated blood sugar levels taken, in order to detect the presence of an insulin-producing beta cell adenoma, the only "functional" islet cell tumor known to exist at that time. This patient, however, had no evidence of hypoglycemia, the lowest fasting blood sugar level being 78 mg%.

After receiving Dr. Jenkins' letter, we were mainly concerned with establishing the presence of a "functioning" insulin-producing tumor, but to no avail. A 15-hour fast did not result in hypoglycemia, and fasting blood sugar levels or four different occasions of 80, 78, 85 and 91 mg%, did not meet the requirements of Whipple's Triad. During the fast for the blood sugar determinations, the patient's symptoms were markedly increased, and she required narcotics for the control of pain. Because her symptoms suggested an impending perforation, emergency gastrointestinal study was done on the last day of the fast. This demonstrated esophagitis, a gastroesophageal ulceration as well as a penetrating

TELEPHONE: DORCHESTER 3-5411

HILGER PERRY JENKINS, M. D.
WOODLAWN CLINIC BUILDING
WOODLAWN HOSPITAL
826 EAST 61ST STREET
CHICAGO 37, ILL.

August 5, 1954.

Robert M. Zollinger, M.D.
Ohio State University,
University Hospital. Dep't. of Surgery,
Columbus, 10, Ohio.

Dear Dr. Zollinger:

I have your letter of July 30th. Your case of primary jejunal ulcer intrigues me very much. Would you be kind enough to send the film on to Dr. Saunders of the American College of Surgeons and we will take a look at it even if you do not have any titles or final editing at the present time. It will be carefully guarded and returned to you with any suggestions which we might offer.

This reminds me a bit of a case that I had of multiple gastric, duodenal and jejunal ulcerations and ultimate perforations in a lady that had an islet tumor of the pancreas. She apparently was carrying out a constant insulin test on her gastro-duodenal-jejunal mechanism which was her undoing. Is there any possibi ity that your little girl has a touch of hyper insulinism as an etiology for this interesting condition.

This sounds like the kind of case we would like to have for the spectacular lesion program. I will look forward to seeing this at your earliest convenience.

Sincerely yours,

Hilger Perry Jenkins
H. P. Jenkins, M.D.

HPJ/ca

CC- H. P. Saunders, M.D.

Figure 7. A copy of the letter from Dr. Hilger Jenkins reminiscing about a patient with multiple ulcerations and perforations associated with an islet cell tumor. He suggests hyperinsulinism as the etiology of this interesting condition.

stomal ulcer at the gastrojejunal junction. The patient was discharged on September 25, to be admitted for possible total gastrectomy within a month.

The patient was hospitalized again on October 17, for the sixth time within a nine-month period, because of ulcer pain which was almost continuous and vomiting which occurred daily. Her four-hour glucose tolerance test was again within normal limits. The urinary steroids showed slight elevation on occasion and her hirsutism was extensive. A repeat Hollander test resulted in an increased acidity, greater than 20 clinical units, suggesting that she had persistently functioning vagal fibers.

Total gastrectomy was carried out on November 3, 1954. A penetrating esophageal ulcer proximal to the cardia was found, and a large ulcer which had practically replaced the posterior side of the gastroduodenal anastomosis was verified. A direct end-to-end anastomosis was made between a Roux-en-Y arm of jejunum (Fig. 5) and the end of the very thickened and inflamed esophagus. The adrenal glands were explored, but no tumor was found; however, a generous biopsy of the left adrenal was taken. Then, because of Dr. Jenkins' suggestions, the pancreas was thoroughly explored before closure for evidence of an insulin-producing tumor. Two small nodules, thought to be lymph nodes, were excised from the anterior aspect of the left side of the body of the pancreas. Examination of the small excised gastric pouch showed prominent rugal folds, and a 1×4 cm ulcer was noted at the esophagogastric junction. The esophagus itself was very thick and indurated, feeling almost like cartilage. The gastroduodenal ulcer measured 4×3 cm.

Microscopic examination of the two nodules removed from the tail of the pancreas showed acinar masses of cuboidal to cylindrical cells which showed irregularly oval nuclei containing finely diffused chromatin and one stellar round-to-oval nucleus. It was also noted that the tumor was markedly demarcated from the normal pancreas by a thin, capsule-like layer of stroma which, in several places, was penetrated by tumor cells. The second and smaller nodule proved to be a lymph node which contained similar types of cells. It was considered to be representative of a metastatic islet cell tumor. Obviously the adenoma was presenting just beneath the capsule of the pancreas.

The patient was discharged on her fifteenth postoperative day but gradually developed symptoms of a stricture at the esophagojejunal junction for which an initial dilatation was performed on January 10, 1955. Following one of these dilatations, she developed substernal pain and had to be admitted to the hospital because of perforation, presumably at the anastomosis, into the right pleural space. Posterior thoracotomy drainage was accomplished, but eventually an empyema on the right side required surgical drainage. The patient then did well and continued to gain weight after surgery; and, as a matter of fact, is still living in her seventeenth postoperative year.

Since this patient was accused of having a functional tumor, her serum was tested for the presence of some undetermined ulcerogenic factor, possibly glucagon. Dr. Ellison carried out a number of studies to test this hypothesis by electrophoretic isolation. An abnormal protein with electrophoretic properties similar to glucagon was isolated from the serum of the living patient; however, this finding could not be reproduced.

At the time of the original presentation, additional cases were reported in the discussions by Dr. Hilger P. Jenkins, Dr. Allen O. Whipple, Dr. Lester Dragstedt, Dr. Edgar Poth, and Dr. Carl E. Moyer. These individuals did not appear to be adverse to accepting the hypothesis that there was a definite relationship between these small, non-specific islet cell tumors and the fulminating ulcer diathesis of the two patients described. In closing the discussion, the senior author noted:

> We have hardly dared to suggest that a relationship might exist between the pancreas and the every-day peptic ulcer. However, the possibility of a pancreatic hormone playing a role in gastric hypersecretion opens up many avenues for experimental and clinical investigation. Certainly the pancreas should be explored in every ulcer patient subjected to surgery, and resection of the body and tail of the pancreas may well be justified before subjecting the rare problem case to total gastrectomy in an effort to control the acid factor.
>
> If these observations accomplish nothing more than a renewal of interest in the ulcer problem with new avenues of study, we will feel justified in reporting these two cases.

Seventeen years later, it is difficult, if not impossible, to relate accurately the development of the concept that certain non-beta islet cell tumors of the pancreas could be implicated in a fulminating ulcer diathesis.

The senior author's special interest in gastropancreatic relationships can be dated to 1947, when a patient was treated who had developed a marginal ulcer after posterior gastroenterostomy. A vagotomy was performed and a large mass involving the body and tail of the pancreas was found, from which a biopsy was taken. The pathologist reported a frozen section diagnosis of "chronic pancreatitis," and accordingly, nothing more was done.

Considerable excitement was generated among the surgical residents when postoperative gastric analyses showed that this lady's acid values were not altered by vagotomy. The implication was that the new professor, fresh from the Army Hospitals of France, was unable to perform a complete vagotomy. In addition, what had been reported as "chronic pancreatitis" was determined on permanent sections to be adenocarcinoma (sic) of the pancreas. Within ten days, the patient was reexplored and the tumor removed. She promptly became achlorhydric and in her five remaining years of life was free of ulcer symptoms. Interestingly enough, a basophile adenoma of the pituitary gland was found at the time of postmortem examination.

This patient's gastric acid values promptly came down and remained normal after removal of the pancreatic tumor, but the true significance of this observation was not appreciated until several years later. It is fair to state that she was my first case of what would later be called the Zollinger-Ellison syndrome.

Surgical physiologists, likewise, had long linked the pancreas with the experimental production of peptic ulcerations. Exalto[720] in 1911, and later in 1923, Mann and Williamson[721] at the Mayo Clinic in their classic experiments demonstrated that isolation of the duodenum and drainage of its secretions into the lower intestine regularly produced chronic progressive ulceration in animals. They attributed this to diversion of the alkaline bile and pancreatic secretions from the first portion of the intestine which first receives the acid gastric contents. Dragstedt,[722] as well as

Ellman and Hartman,[724] confirmed this finding in 1930, using dogs with an external fistula. This explanation, however, came into question when Mann showed that ulcers still occurred even when secretions from the isolated duodenum were diverted into the upper part of the stomach, so that complete mixing of the gastric contents occurred. Then, in 1942, Dragstedt[728] reported that the incidence of experimental ulcer following external pancreatic fistulas was almost 100 per cent, but after ligation of the pancreatic duct was 29 per cent, and only 1.3 per cent following pancreatectomy.

It was Poth in 1948[730] who raised the questions: Is this paradox real or apparent? Does the pancreas have an intrinsic influence upon ulcer formation other than that of mere alteration of the pH of the duodenal contents? He injected a series of dogs with histamine-in-beeswax, using the method developed by Varco and Wangensteen[729] after total pancreatectomy, after ligation of the pancreatic ducts, and after producing diabetes with Alloxan®. Fulminating ulcerations developed when the pancreatic secretions were diverted from the duodenum. While pancreatectomy itself did not seem to produce ulcers, the result of histamine stimulation seemed to suggest a strong predisposition to ulcer formation after extirpation of the gland. That diabetes might prove to be an inhibitory effect on ulcer formation was not proved in these experiments. Poth (Fig. 8) then concluded that "both the internal and external secretions of the pancreas may be implicated in ulcer formation," and in further experiments suggested that the endocrine portion of the pancreas, apart from its well-known role in producing insulin, probably elaborates another hormone which could directly influence gastric function (Fig. 9).

As the available clinical literature was reviewed, it was obvious that additional case reports had been written which pointed out the association of peptic ulcer and "non-functioning" islet cell tumors, but the association was regarded as coincidental. For many years, islet cell tumors were generally considered to be "non-functioning" if they did not produce insulin. Brown, Neville, and Hazard,[731] of the Cleveland Clinic, described a patient in 1950 as having an islet cell adenoma, without hypoglycemia, causing

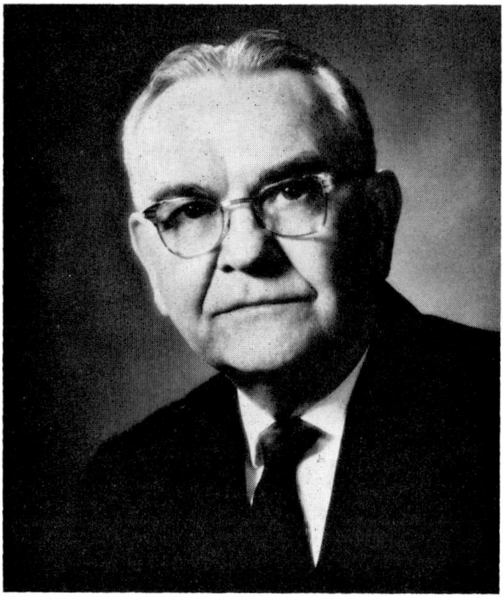

Figure 8. Dr. Edgar J. Poth, Professor of Surgery, University of Texas, Galveston, who in 1948 suggested that both the external as well as the internal secretions of the pancreas may be involved in the etiology of an ulcer.

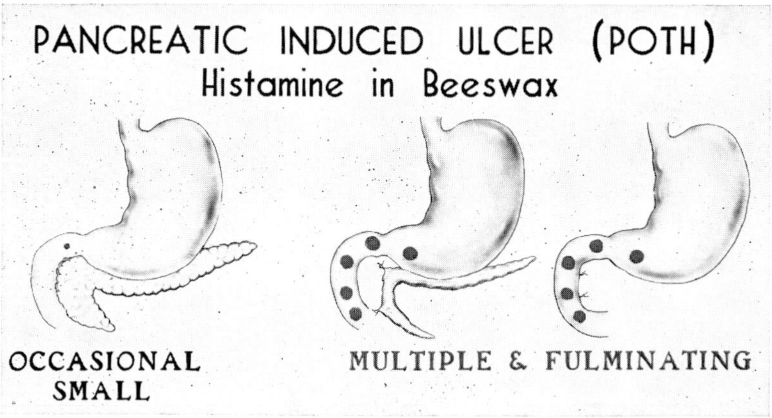

Figure 9. A schematic drawing of the experiments by Dr. Edgar J. Poth of the University of Texas involving the production of histamine-induced ulcers following ligation of the pancreatic ducts as well as pancreatectomy. He concluded "that both the internal and external secretions of the pancreas may be implicated in ulcer formation."

duodenal obstruction. Their patient had gastric hypersecretion by Ewald test meal, and diarrhea but no ulcer. The patient had complete remission of symptoms after local excision of the tumor. Janowitz and Crohn,[732] in 1951, had described the "extremely rare occurrence of duodenal ulcer and hyperinsulinism due to an adenoma of the islands of Langerhans." Surgical cure of the hypoglycemia, effected by removal of the pancreatic tumor, had no mitigating effect on the clinical course of the patient's duodenal ulcer. The late Roar Strom of Norway,[734] in 1952, had reported a case of insuloma, consisting of atypical beta cells, associated with chronic peptic ulcer which had required three surgical operations within three years and finally was cured after resection of an 8 gram tumor from the tail of the pancreas. He suggested that there might be a possible relationship between the tumor and the increased peptic acidity, but in concluding his article, stated that "no observations indicate that hypoglycemic insulinomas are apt to dispose to peptic ulcer formation. *The simultaneous occurrence of insuloma in peptic ulcer is thus probably not a causal coincidence.*"

Before the description of the ulcerogenic tumor syndrome, attention had been called to the occasional association of islet cell tumors with adenomas of the parathyroid or pituitary glands, leading to the designation of "adenomatosis." Underdahl, in 1953,[735] reviewed 14 such cases in which a pituitary tumor, islet cell adenomas, and parathyroid tumors, or a combination of two of these, occurred in the same patient. In addition to this review of the literature, they added eight additional cases of this syndrome which had been encountered at the Mayo Clinic. Parathyroid tumors were present in all; pituitary tumors in four, or half of these cases; and five had islet cell tumors. They called attention to the multiplicity of the tumors as a striking feature which occurred both in relation to the parathyroids and to the pancreatic islets. Wermer (Fig. 10), in his classic presentation entitled "Genetic Aspects of Adenomatosis of Endocrine Glands,"[736] pointed out that the simultaneous occurrence of adenomas of the anterior pituitary and the parathyroids, and islet cell tumors in one individual had been known as a pathologic rarity for many years, going back to the original description by Erdheim in

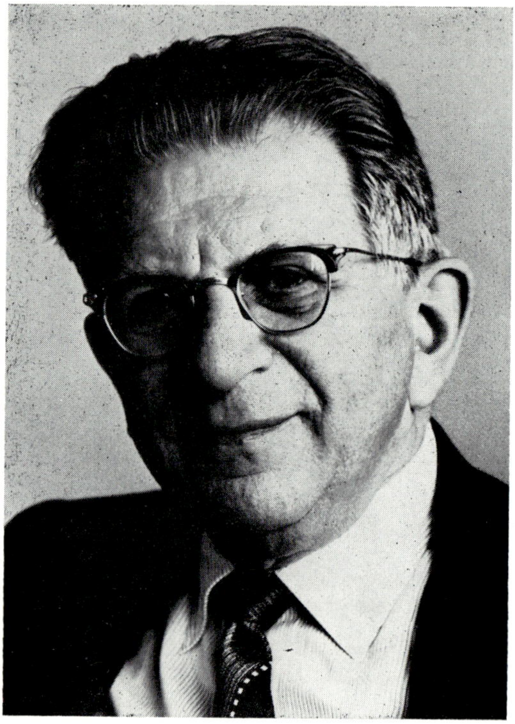

Figure 10. Dr. Paul Wermer described a syndrome of familial multiple endocrine adenomatoses in which peptic ulcer was a prominent feature. He believed it was caused by a dominant autosomal gene with a high degree of penetrance.

1903.[716] Wermer presented a family in whom the syndrome of multiple endocrine adenomas had occurred in several members of two generations. He called attention to certain lesions in non-endocrine organs, i.e. peptic ulcerations, which are frequently found in the same patients and which belonged to the total syndrome. Wermer stated in 1954 "that the syndrome in this family was caused by a dominant autosomal gene with a high degree of penetrance, that the gross and microscopic findings in the pancreas were different from those seen in the more common, single adenomas and that peptic ulcers of the stomach and duodenum were frequently found in such patients, but that they were merely another expression of the abnormal gene."

1955-1960: THE ERA OF CHALLENGE

From the original report of the ulcerogenic tumor syndrome came a chain reaction of further case reports from all over the world, and in 1956, Eiseman (Fig. 11) and Maynard suggested characterizing this diagnostic triad under the eponym Zollinger-Ellison syndrome.[2] In 1956 again, Dr. Ellison was able to collect a total of 24 published cases with an additional five obtained from a review of 1,500 autopsy reports of patients who died in The Ohio State University Hospitals.[3] As a matter of fact, most of the publications before 1960 were culled from postmortem material, and many of these cases were discovered by reviewing pathological files, after the stimulus of the original publication. While the existence of the syndrome could be supported by the

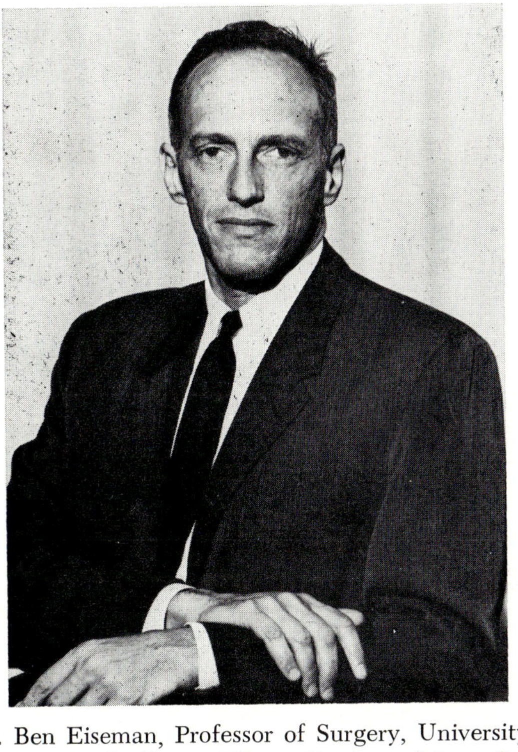

Figure 11. Dr. Ben Eiseman, Professor of Surgery, University of Colorado, who coined the phrase "Zollinger-Ellison Syndrome" in a discussion of the paper of Dr. Ellison's before the Society of University Surgeons in 1956.

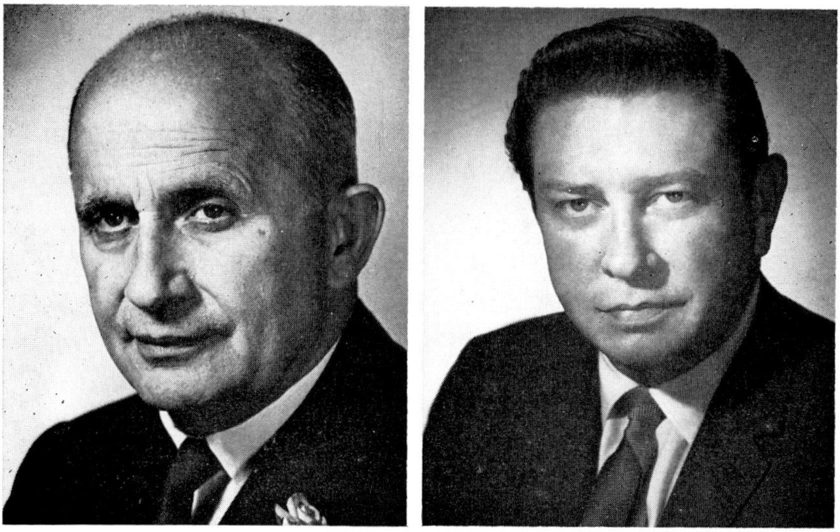

Figure 12. Robert M. Zollinger and Edwin H. Ellison, who presented the concept of the ulcerogenic tumor syndrome in 1955 with a report of two cases.

increasing number of case reports, failure to identify the postulated humoral mechanism and the islet cell of origin led many authors to alternative conclusions.

In addition to the observations by Poth and by Eiseman which disproved that glucagon was the offending hormone, Waddell and associates[43] studied in considerable detail two patients having the ulcerogenic syndrome. They said "it is not true that pancreatic abnormalities are an essential feature of the disease." In support of their conclusion, they suggested that "many aspects of the abnormal gastric secretory process were consistent with the concept of hypersecretion resulting from an autonomic dysfunction"; that "hypothalamic dysfunction might produce unusual autonomic activity and through its influence on the pituitary gland account for multiple endocrine gland anomalies such as those observed in patients with the Zollinger-Ellison syndrome."

Donaldson and colleagues[7] reported a patient who had extreme gastric hypersecretion for two years before recognized clinical manifestations of peptic ulceration occurred. This experience, combined with the fact that 6 of the 21 cases they reviewed had multiple endocrine abnormalities, suggested that factors other than those of pancreatic origin might be responsible for the syndrome. They believed that the nature of the relationship between peptic ulcer and multiple endocrine tumors was obscure and raised the question that one or several of the endocrine tumors might be responsible for the development of peptic ulceration and that some as-yet-unknown mechanism was the common cause of both the peptic ulcer and the endocrine tumors.

Rudolf, Dammin, and Moore, in a presentation before the Society of University Surgeons in 1960, proposed the hypothesis that there had been a relative or absolute failure of secretion of one of the target endocrine organs.[80] They concluded, "This, in turn, has brought about hyperplasia and in some cases, adenomatous changes in amphophill and basophil cells of the pituitary. These changes are reflected in an increased production of one or more of the trophic hormones. Those, in turn, cause hyperplasias

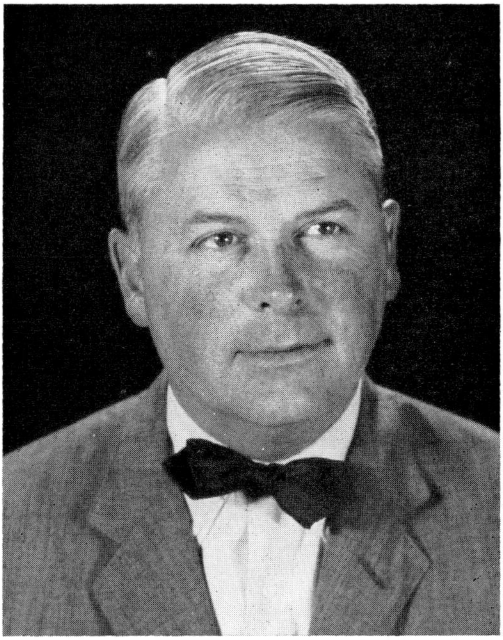

Figure 13. Dr. Melvin Osborne, Associate Professor, Department of Surgery, Harvard University School of Medicine, whose saline extract of an islet cell tumor demonstrated, in 1961, the presence of a gastric secretagogue.

or adenomas of the other target endocrine organs. The acid-peptic axis is stimulated directly, through parietal cell hyperplasia, or indirectly, as a byproduct of secretion of the adrenals, gonads or parathyroids. Intractable ulceration results."

THE UNIVERSITY OF LIVERPOOL

TELEPHONE ROYAL 6022

HAEC OTIA STUDIA FOVENT

FROM THE
PROFESSOR OF PHYSIOLOGY

May 5th 1960

MAY 10 1960
DEPARTMENT OF SURGERY

Dear Doctor Zollinger,

You will probably remember my visit last Spring to Dr. Ogden's Department in your University; I have thought many times with pleasure of our meeting and all-too-brief discussion of the Zollinger-Ellison syndrome. I am writing now to give you news of this which I think will interest you. A few weeks ago a case appeared in Birmingham, inwhich the only pathology found at operation was a small tumour in the pancreas, which was removed, with relief of the symptoms. My colleague Dr. Hilda Tracy and I were fortunate enough to obtain a portion of the tumour. From this we made extracts by a method we have recently evolved for the extraction from hog antral mucosa of the hormone gastrin (Journal of Physiology, 1959, Proceedings of November meeting). The tumour extracts were injected into conscious pouch dogs (2); in each case they caused a large and prolonged secretory response, identical in character with that produced in the same animals by the injection of a gastrin extract made from hog antral mucosa. The gastrin-like activity present in the tumour was equivalent to that present in 33-45 times its weight of hog antral mucosa. The tumour extract was shown not to contain either histamine or insulin.

Our report on these experiments is now in press in "The Lancet"; it should appear in two or three weeks.

I do not know whether you are likely to visit Europe in the near future, but if you do, it will give us the greatest pleasure to welcome you to Liverpool. Please give my warmest regards to Dr. Ogden.

With all good wishes,

Yours ever,

R. A. Gregory.

R. A. Gregory

Professor R. M. Zollinger,
Department of Surgery,
The University,
Columbus, Ohio, U.S.A.

Figure 14. A letter of May 5, 1960, from Professor R. A. Gregory of the University of Liverpool relating to his exciting findings that tumor extracts were similar to extracts of hog antral mucosa for gastrin activity equivalent to 33 to 45 times its weight of hog antral mucosa.

Since the original postulated gastric secretagogue of islet cell origin had not as yet been identified and the supposition that glucagon might be responsible had not been substantiated, the report of Osborn (Fig. 13) and colleagues in 1960 was particularly significant. They carried out studies of the extraction of a possible gastric secretagogue[75] from an ulcerogenic islet cell tumor. The authors utilized slightly over 2 gm of pancreatic islet cell carcinoma to make a saline extract. It had been kept frozen for two years. They reported that this extract stimulated acid secretion from a vagotomized, isolated Heidenhain pouch of a dog when given intravenously. They also concluded that "from the limited data available, it appears that the substance called N-1 resists prolonged freezing at ordinary freezer temperatures; tolerates postmortem autolysis to some extent, and is soluble in water and can pass through a cellophane membrane slowly when dialyzed; is not identified with histamine, glucagon, or insulin, quickly affects acid secretion from a Heidenhain pouch for a short time when given intravenously, and is not present in control preparations made from human liver and pancreas."

In a letter dated May 6, 1960, from Professor R. A. Gregory, University of Liverpool, we learned that he and Dr. Hilda Tracy had been able to obtain gastrin-like activity from an extract of an islet cell tumor which was equivalent to that present in 35 to 45 times its weight of hog antral mucosa (Fig. 14).

The culmination of the abundant literature dealing with one or

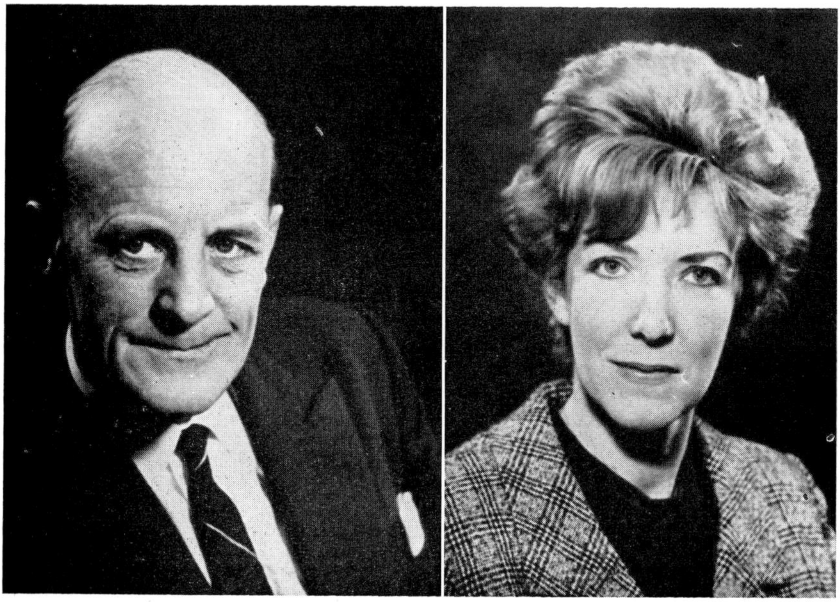

Figure 15. Professor R. A. Gregory and Professor Hilda Tracy of the Department of Physiology, University of Liverpool, England, in 1960, confirmed that the gastric secretagogue of the ulcerogenic tumor was indeed similar to gastrin.

another aspect of this syndrome and the various etiological theories was Gregory and Tracy's achievement in 1961 demonstrating the hormonal nature of the secretagogue as "gastrin-like" (Fig. 15). A specimen of cherry-sized tumor had been made available by Professor Stammers and colleagues of Birmingham, England, through Dr. Wilfred Sircus of Edinburgh (Fig. 16). By the picric acid extraction they used to secure gastrin from hog antral mucosa, they extracted a substance with the same secretagogue properties as gastrin, in amounts, weight for weight, 35 to 45 times greater (Fig. 17).

THE ERA OF CONFIRMATION

After the initial identification of gastrin as the ulcerogenic hormone elaborated by non-beta islet cell tumors, there was an avalanche of publications regarding this polypeptide. In 1961, Grossman (Fig. 18), Tracy and Gregory extracted the tumor which was sent to them by Marks, and a gastrin-like secretagogue was obtained from both the primary tumor as well as the hepatic

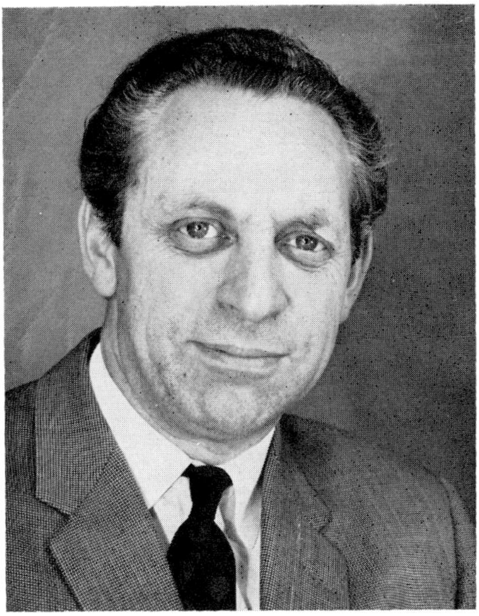

Figure 16. Dr. Wilfred Sircus of Edinburgh, whose investigations of the ulcerogenic and diarrheagenic tumor syndromes have been significant.

Reprinted from THE LANCET, *May* 14, 1960, *pp.* 1045–1048

EXTRACTION OF A GASTRIN-LIKE SUBSTANCE FROM A PANCREATIC TUMOUR IN A CASE OF ZOLLINGER-ELLISON SYNDROME

R. A. GREGORY
D.Sc. Lond., Ph.D., M.R.C.S.
GEORGE HOLT PROFESSOR OF PHYSIOLOGY

HILDA J. TRACY
M.B. Lpool
ASSISTANT LECTURER

DEPARTMENT OF PHYSIOLOGY, UNIVERSITY OF LIVERPOOL

J. M. FRENCH
M.D., Ph.D. Birm., M.R.C.P.
MEMBER OF EXTERNAL STAFF, MEDICAL RESEARCH COUNCIL; MACKENZIE-MACKINNON RESEARCH FELLOW, DEPARTMENT OF MEDICINE, UNIVERSITY OF BIRMINGHAM

W. SIRCUS
M.D. Lpool, Ph.D. Sheff., M.R.C.P.E., M.R.C.P.
MEMBER OF EXTERNAL STAFF, MEDICAL RESEARCH COUNCIL; LECTURER AND PHYSICIAN, DEPARTMENT OF MEDICINE, UNIVERSITY OF EDINBURGH, AND GASTRO-INTESTINAL UNIT, WESTERN GENERAL HOSPITAL

Figure 17. The title of the original paper of Gregory, Tracy, French, *et al.*, which appeared in *Lancet,* May 14, 1960. The publication announcing the extraction of a gastrin-like substance from the islet cell tumor of the pancreas associated with a fulminating ulcer diathesis.

metastases. Code and colleagues, in 1962,[138] were able to extract a gastrin-like substance by an acid-acetone technic, after conservation in picric acid. From three cases of the ulcerogenic syndrome, they were able to extract a gastric secretagogue from both the primary and metastatic tumors. A parathyroid tumor and normal parathyroid tissue from the same patient were similarly extracted but exhibited no activity. Davis, also in 1962,[142] found gastrin in

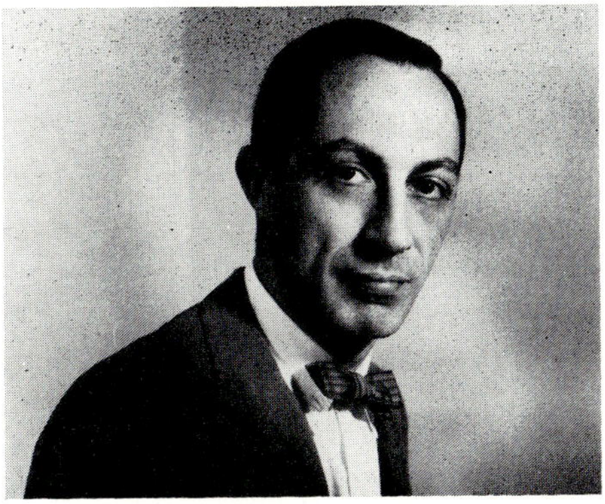

Figure 18. Professor Morton Grossman of the University of California, Los Angeles, whose many fundamental contributions in gastrointestinal physiology included the early studies on hormones extracted from islet cell tumors.

the tumors removed from a 15-year-old boy who had the complete syndrome of fulminating ulcer and diarrhea, which was treated by total gastrectomy. Friesen[147] was likewise able to show that metastases have the same kind of activity as the primary tumor or tumors, while a carcinoma of the exocrine pancreas submitted to the same process of extraction provided no active substances. Finally, in April, 1964, Gregory and Tracy[263] published a summary of their previous work with gastrin, together with a method for massive extraction. From porcine antrum they had been able to isolate two almost identical polypeptides which they named Gastrin I and Gastrin II. These authors felt that the identity of these agents with the secretagogue from ulcerogenic islet cell tumors was firmly established: "We showed that the pure natural gastrins had exactly the same range and physiological activities as is possessed by crude extracts from a Zollinger-Ellison tumor and regard this as strong evidence that the active principle of such tumors is, in fact, gastrin."

CLINICAL SPECTRUM OF THE ULCEROGENIC TUMOR SYNDROME

In the 18 years which have elapsed since the ulcerogenic tumor syndrome was first delineated, this disease entity, at first a medical rarity, has assumed increasing importance to surgeons, internists, and physiologists who are called upon to deal with the problems of peptic ulcer. After its introduction in 1955, there were a few case reports in 1956, considerably more in 1960, and between 1964 and 1967, the number doubled, until with additional cases reported in 1971 there were more than 800 case reports available to us for analysis (Fig. 19). [A complete bibliography of the case reports and personal communications can be found beginning on page 79.] This in no way represents the true incidence since the ulcerogenic syndrome has become so well identified that individual case reports are often not submitted for publication. We have maintained a registry of the reported cases as has Wilson of Milwaukee.

The diagnosis of an ulcerogenic tumor is being made earlier, and also more frequently, on the basis of suspicious findings in the patient's clinical history. While no clinical history can yet be described as "classical," the possibility of an ulcerogenic, non-beta islet cell tumor of the pancreas should be considered immediately if:

1. There is a primary ulceration in the jejunum, beyond the ligament of Treitz.

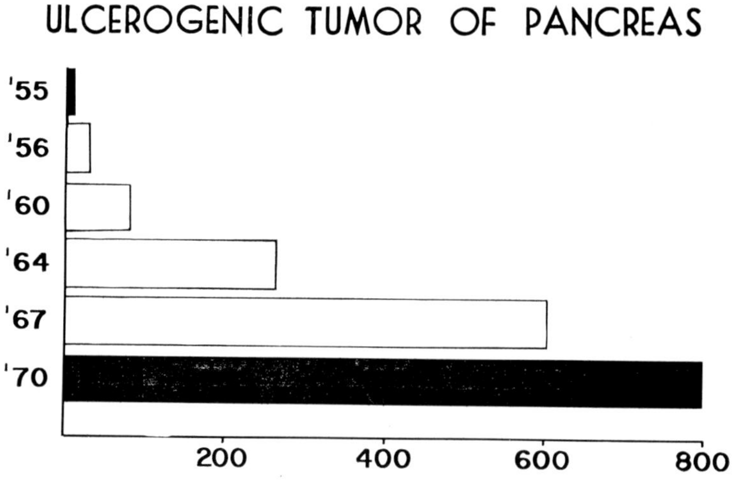

Figure 19. A graph showing the increasing recognition of the islet cell tumor syndrome in the reported cases between 1955 and 1971.

2. A patient with ulcer disease produces 1 L or more of gastric juice in 12 hours from an unobstructed stomach with 100 mEq/L or more of free hydrochloric acid.
3. A fulminating ulcer diathesis occurs for the first time in a patient who is either very young or very old.
4. Severe ulcer symptoms with perforation or hemorrhage occur in the immediate postpartum period or soon after a standard ulcer operation.
5. Severe and persistent diarrhea is accompanied by steatorrhea and massive amounts of gastric secretion, either with or without evidence of a fulminating ulcer diathesis.
6. Ulcer symptoms associated with hypercalcemia or other evidence of polyglandular involvement.

The entire endocrine system as well as the family history of each suspected patient must be thoroughly screened since, as Wermer and others have pointed out, there is a tendency for more than one gland of internal secretion to be involved with the islet cell tumor. This is commonly referred to as multiple endocrine adenomatosis, or the MEA syndrome, with a familial variant which is known as the Wermer syndrome.

On the other hand, the tendency to implicate an ulcerogenic tumor rather than an inadequate or incomplete operation which has not controlled the acid factor may be too great in problem cases of recurrent ulceration. Invariably, a review of a series of recurrent ulcer patients will show that the real problem lies in an overlooked vagus nerve, particularly the posterior one, on inadequate gastric resection without vagotomy; a gastroenterostomy without vagotomy; a gastroenterostomy improperly placed too far to the left, with or without vagotomy, resulting in antral distention; or a retained gastric antrum. Also to be considered are extragastric causes of gastric hypersecretion which have been thoroughly studied by Elliott (Fig. 20) and colleagues,[197] such as chronic calcific pancreatitis, short bowel syndrome, etc.

In an effort to gain more insight into the clinical symptoms of the ulcerogenic tumor syndrome, our registry, containing some 800 case histories, was subjected to computer analysis. The age range in the 800 cases shows that the development of severe ulcer symp-

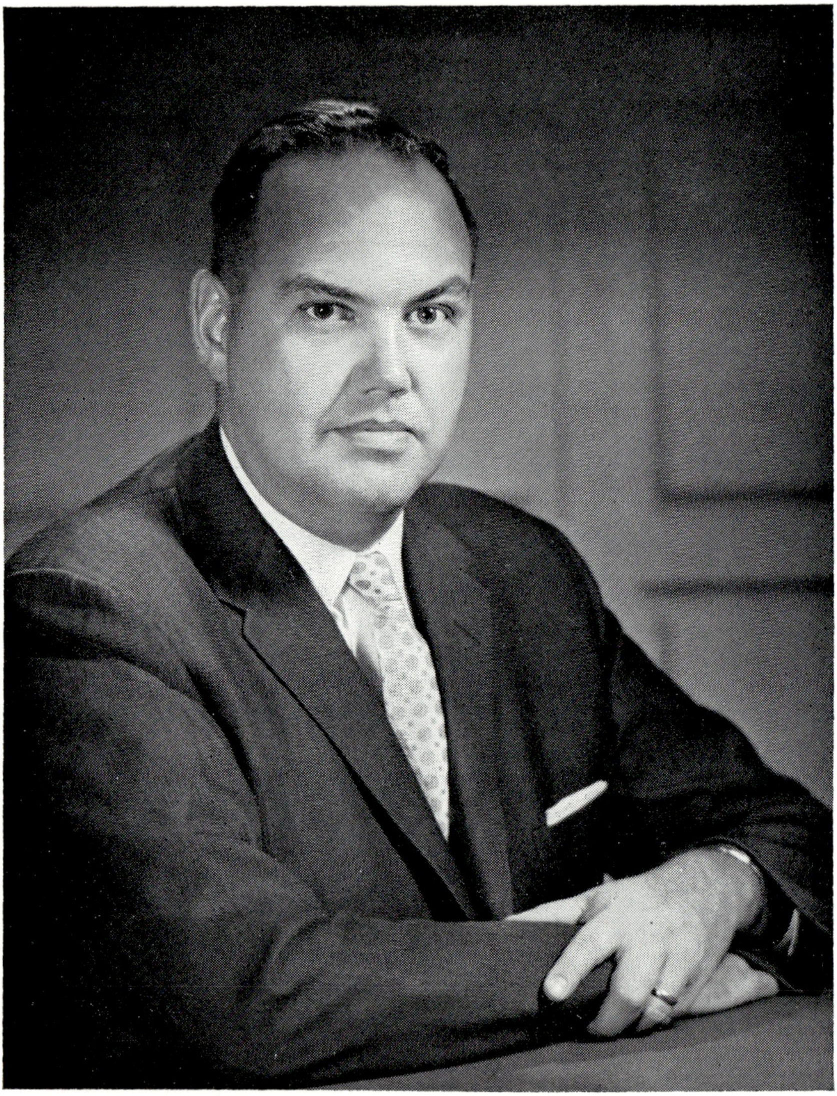

Figure 20. Dr. Daniel W. Elliott, surgical investigator, who has contributed to the better understanding of the hormonal relationship between the pancreas and gastric section.

toms in two extreme age groups, namely under 20 and after 70, strongly implicates the ulcerogenic tumor. In contrast to the ordinary duodenal ulcer patient where the age occurrence is well below 40 years, the peak of the ulcerogenic syndrome appears to be at about 50, with the highest range running between 35 and 60 (Fig. 21). The slow growth of the ulcerogenic tumor is supported by the long history which many patients present before the diagnosis is made. An ulcerogenic tumor should be considered in any woman who develops perforation or a massive hemorrhage from a duodenal ulcer in the postpartum period. Approximately eight cases of this type have been described. The hormones of pregnancy protect these women against ulceration, a finding established by Sandweiss and colleagues in 1938,[726] but immediately after delivery they tend to get into severe difficulty.

The symptomatology of the ulcerogenic syndrome is dominated by the ulcer in more than 90 per cent of the cases; diarrhea is the main feature in the remainder. The common complications associated with the ulcer and the incidence of their occurrence are tabulated in Fig. 22. Forty-three per cent of the patients, or more than 300, had intractability to treatment as a complication requiring surgery. In 32 per cent, hemorrhage was the complication re-

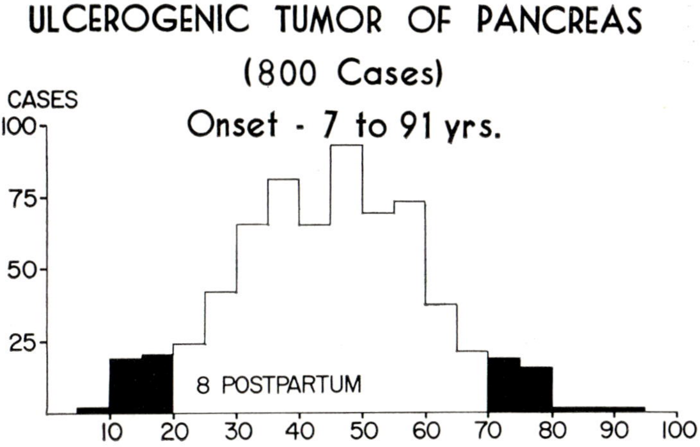

Figure 21. Severe ulcer symptoms which occur in the two age extremes of life or in the immediate postpartum period should make the clinician suspicious of an ulcerogenic tumor of the pancreas.

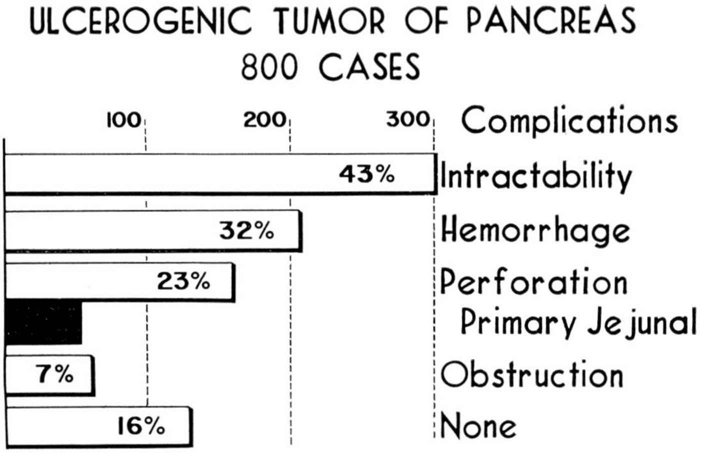

Figure 22. Intractability was the most common and obstruction the least common of the complications in the 800 case histories surveyed. Primary jejunal ulcerations should be considered pathognomonic of ulcerogenic tumor. There were no complications in approximately 16 per cent.

quiring surgery, while in 23 per cent, perforation was the catastrophe which mandated emergency surgical intervention. It is significant that only 7 per cent of the patients had symptoms of obstruction. Perhaps this is related to the fulminating nature of the ulcer diathesis, in contrast to the usual clinical picture of healing then recurrence with scar formation which is seen in the non–ulcerogenic–tumor–type of ulcer patient. In 16 per cent of the patients, there was no particularly serious or unusual complication noted in the history. In this latter group, the diagnosis was either an accidental finding at the time of surgery, usually for ulcer, or all too frequently an unexpected finding at the time of postmortem examination.

It was noted that about 8 per cent of the patients had multiple perforations (Fig. 23-a). Of great significance is the finding that in 6 per cent of this group, the perforation occurred primarily in the jejunum, just beyond the ligament of Treitz. In the original two case reports, jejunal ulcerations had been a prominent finding in the patients' early histories. In our judgment, the finding of an active ulcer or perforated ulcer in the jejunum just beyond the ligament of Treitz in a patient who has had no previous gastric

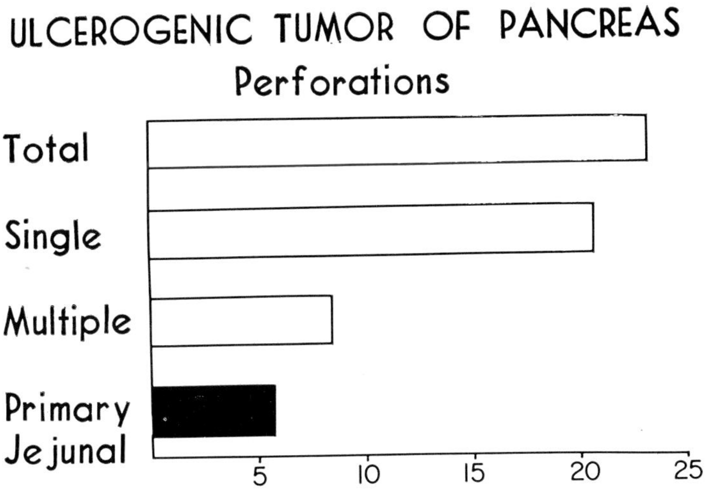

Figure 23-a. Multiple perforations and ulcerations occurring just beyond the ligament of Treitz should strongly suggest the presence of an ulcerogenic tumor.

surgery is almost pathognomonic of an ulcerogenic tumor, whether or not the surgeon is able to find it. It is realized that an increasing number of causes for jejunal ulceration, including various medications must be considered; but this is an ulcer in a very unusual

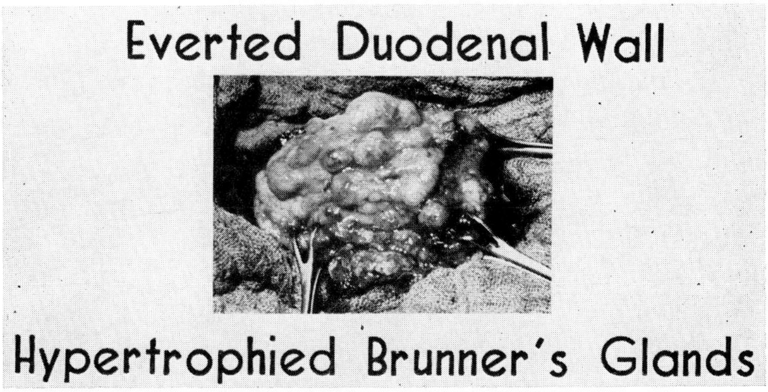

Figure 23-b. The inverted stump of the divided duodenum showing nodularity of the mucosa due to hypertrophied Brunner's glands, a possible secondary effect of marked gastric hypersecretion.

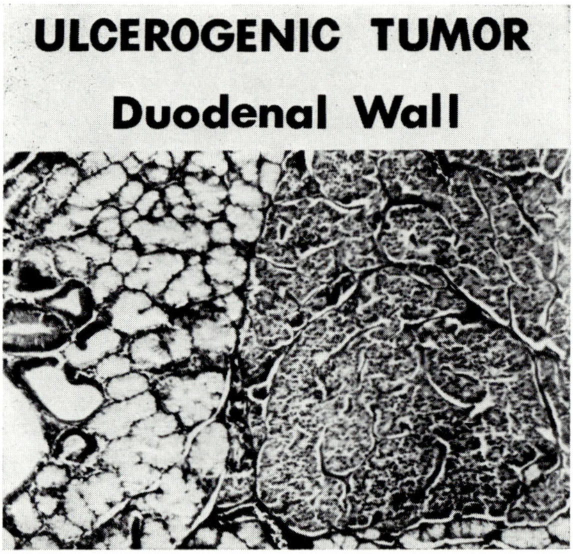

Figure 24. Microscopic sections of the small islet cell tumor in the wall of the duodenum which could not be found at the time of the initial operation. Tumor occurred in the wall of the duodenum in 82 of the 800 reported cases.

location and one to be taken very seriously when found. We have observed a patient who had closure of two previous perforations of the jejunum near the ligament of Treitz, only to have a recurrence for the third time. At the time of the third operation, a thorough search was made for an ulcerogenic tumor, but none could be found. The duodenal mucosa was covered with nodules which proved to be hypertrophied Brunner glands (Fig. 23-b). In the absence of microscopic proof, even though convinced that an ulcerogenic tumor was present, vagotomy hemigastrectomy and Billroth I reconstruction were carried out. A sufficient rim of duodenum was resected to permit microscopic examination, but not until the final sections was a microadenoma found within the wall of the duodenum (Fig. 24). Within one year, this patient had developed recurrent ulcer symptoms which required total gastrectomy.

A possible explanation for the reason why duodenal ulcer may not occur when there is an ulceration in the jejunum beyond the ligament of Treitz has been schematically outlined in Figure 25. Attention is called to the increased size of the duodenum with its thick wall and dual blood supply along the inner curvature. The duodenum is also protected by alkaline secretions from the bile and pancreatic juice. As the large volume of hydrochloric acid are "jet propelled" from the third portion of the duodenum around the ligament of Treitz, they come in contact with the thin-walled jejunum which has a relatively poor blood supply by comparison. While the cause is not certain, this mechanical theory is offered as a possible rational explanation.

Although present in one of the original patients, diarrhea was not emphasized in the clinical syndrome because we had held to the triad concept as popularized by Whipple.[727] It became obvious in a relatively short period of time, however, that the syndrome should have been extended to include diarrhea. A review of the more than 800 cases of ulcerogenic tumor of the pancreas clearly shows that diarrhea or steatorrhea may be associated with a fulminating ulcer diathesis in about 30 per cent of the patients, while in an additional 6 per cent, there is a severe diarrhea associated with marked gastric hypersecretion, but without duodenal or je-

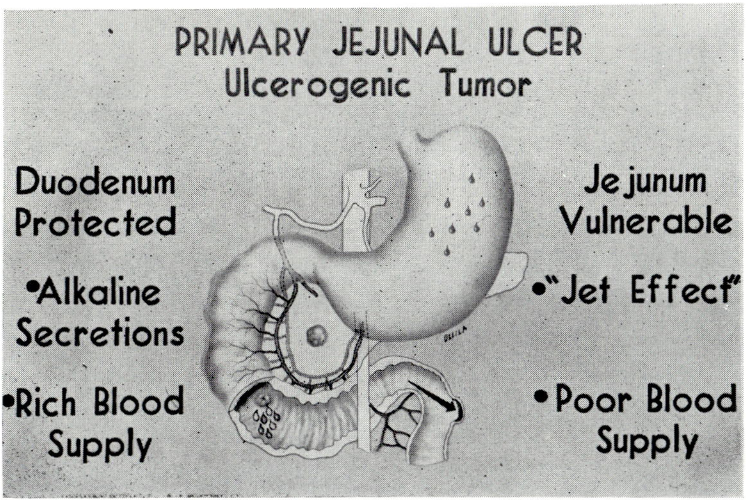

Figure 25. A diagram with the suggested explanation for the occurrence of a primary jejunal ulcer just beyond the ligament of Treitz.

junal ulcerations (Fig. 26). This diarrhea has been explained on the basis of the excessive gastric acid secretion, resulting in irritation of the duodenum and small intestine as well as bringing about neutralization of the alkaline secretions of the pancreas and bile, leading to steatorrhea (Fig. 27). As soon as the tumor and metastases had been identified as producing gastrin, it was realized that this hormone had the potential to produce increased gastrointestinal motility which no doubt would also contribute to the relatively high incidence of associated diarrhea. Triple lumen tube perfusion studies of the jejunum in several patients with ulcerogenic tumors revealed an increased volume of fluid in the upper jejunum, even though the excessive gastric juice had been aspirated.[669] It was suggested that the diarrhea may be caused by direct inhibition of jejunal absorption through mechanisms in addition to, and independent of, the action of tumor-elaborated gastrin on gastric acid production.

As mentioned, the MEA and Wermer syndromes had been established before the ulcerogenic syndrome was described. In at

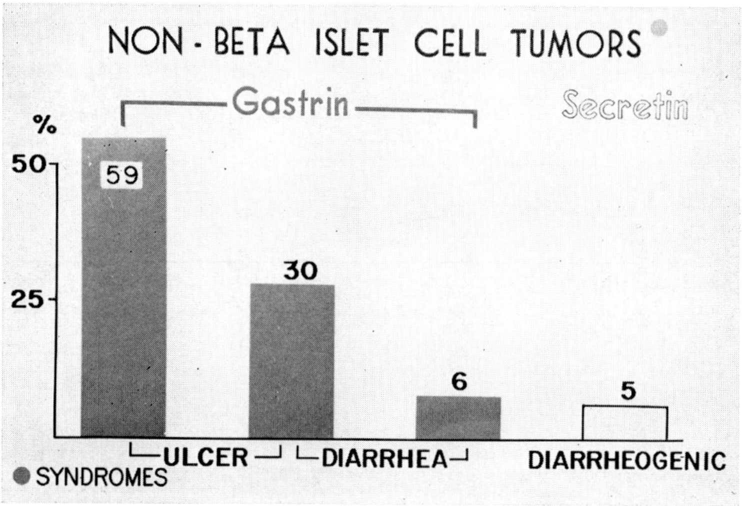

Figure 26. Diarrhea is commonly associated with the ulcerogenic islet cell tumor syndrome with or without associated ulcer formation. In approximately 5 per cent of the patients, an islet cell tumor is associated with achlorhydria and a severe watery diarrhea.

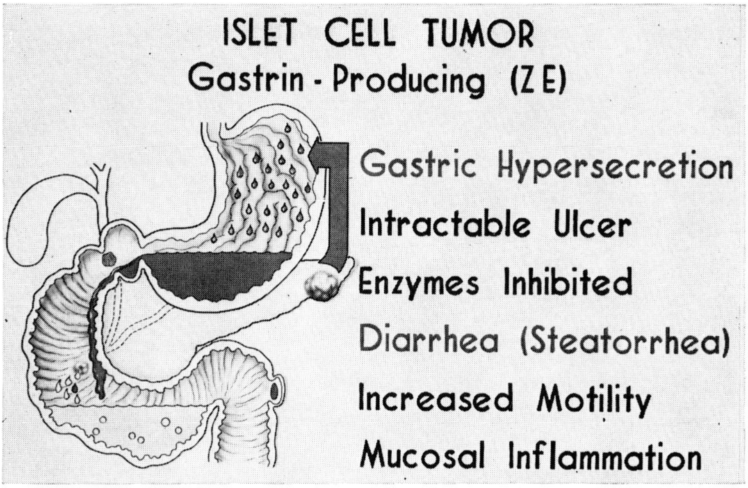

Figure 27. A schematic drawing demonstrating some of the factors responsible for the steatorrhea associated with marked gastric hypersecretion. In addition, the polypeptide gastrin alters the transport of the gastrointestinal secretions.

least half of our 800 cases, there was no specific mention made as to whether or not the possibility of associated endocrine adenomata had been studied. Pituitary tumors were present in 10 per cent of the cases, parathyroid adenomas in 22 per cent, thyroid adenomas in 10 per cent, adrenal adenomas in 13 per cent, beta cell adenomas and carcinoid tumors in 2 per cent (Fig. 28). These statistics can only be accepted as approximate because of the lack of details in so many of the case reports; however, they appear to be consistent with the observations of Ellison and Wilson,[255] who found a rather consistent rate of associated MEA in about 20 per cent of the patients. In contrast, the Wermer's Syndrome was noted in approximately 5 per cent of our cases. These data clearly support the wisdom of a complete endocrine survey, when time permits, in any patient suspected of harboring an ulcerogenic tumor of the pancreas.

Tumors occur in all age groups, and islet cell tumors are no exception. In the 800 cases studied, 0.6 per cent were under 10 years of age and 4.5 per cent were between 10 and 16 years of age. Because of the unknown response of children to total gastrectomy

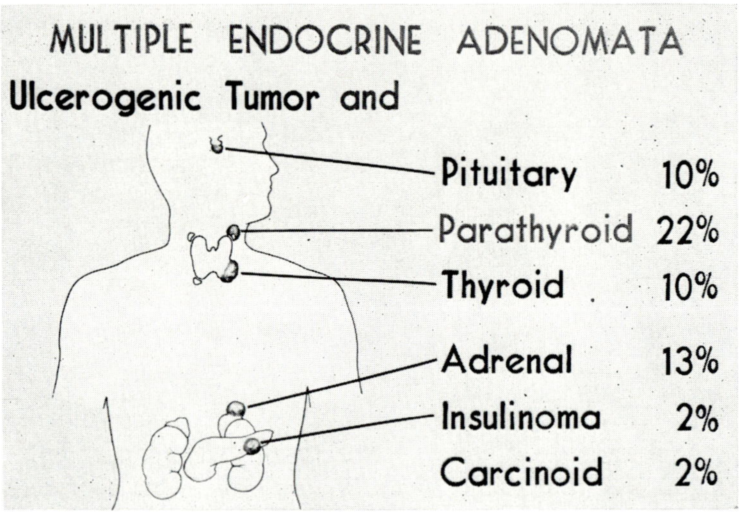

Figure 28. A second adenoma of a gland of internal secretion occurs in approximately 20 per cent of the patients with an islet cell tumor. Involvements of the parathyroid are by far the most common and this may well be a secondary effect of the syndrome.

for proven islet cell tumors, Wilson and Ellison in 1965[347] evaluated the reported cases in the literature as well as their experiences with one patient. At that time, 300 case reports of ulcerogenic tumor were studied with eight children having undergone gastric resections for an ulcerogenic tumor. The ages varied between 8 and 15 years. All of the children had bleeding as their major complaints. Seven of the eight patients at operation had evidence of metastases from the islet cell tumor, while one exhibited only islet cell hyperplasia. The children who underwent total gastrectomy were living at the time of the report, while those with less than a total gastrectomy had died. The authors pointed out that these youngsters did surprisingly well after total gastrectomy, with either a slowdown or regression of the metastases. Five years later, in 1971, Wilson, Schulte, and Meade reported on 15 cases collected from their tumor registry.[709] Of the eight children who had had less than a total gastrectomy, six were dead (Fig. 29). All seven children with total gastrectomy had remained alive and well, despite the fact that they all had metastases and/or

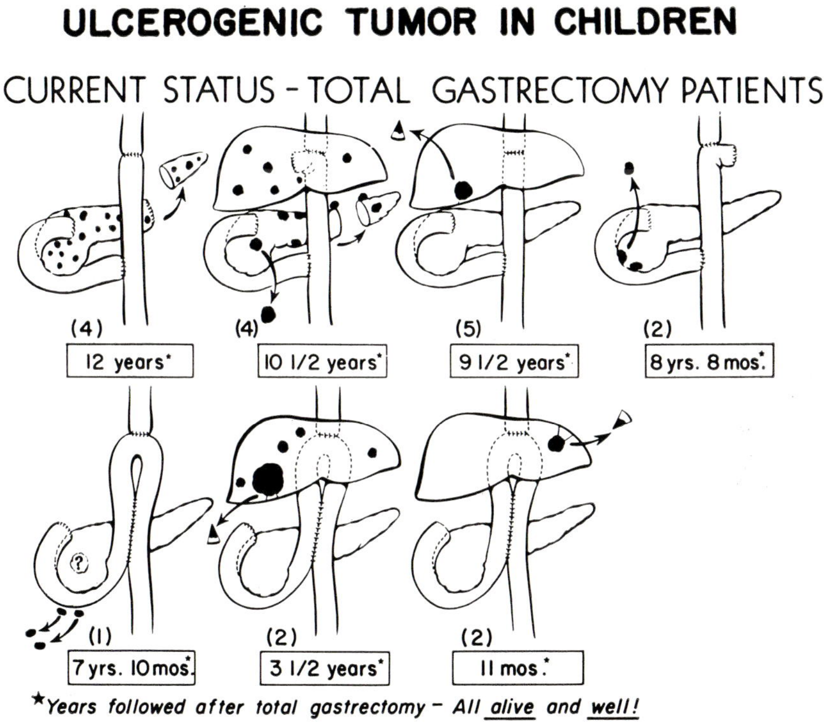

Figure 29. Study by Stuart Wilson *et al.*, indicating the disasterous effect of less than total gastric resection in the treatment of an islet cell tumor in children.

multiple tumors at the time of operation (Fig. 30). These investigators had the unusual opportunity of carrying out serial bioassay and immunoassay determinations for gastrin in six of the seven patients for periods as long as 5 to 11 years after the total gastrectomy. In one patient, the gastrin level had been elevated for six years, but had fallen to low levels after eight years. In two other patients, the gastrin levels progressively decreased each year following total gastrectomy, which would seem to indicate that the metastatic tumors had regressed.

DIAGNOSIS OF THE ULCEROGENIC TUMOR SYNDROME

The patient with an ulcerogenic tumor of the pancreas will commonly have such a gigantic hypersecretion that dehydration and

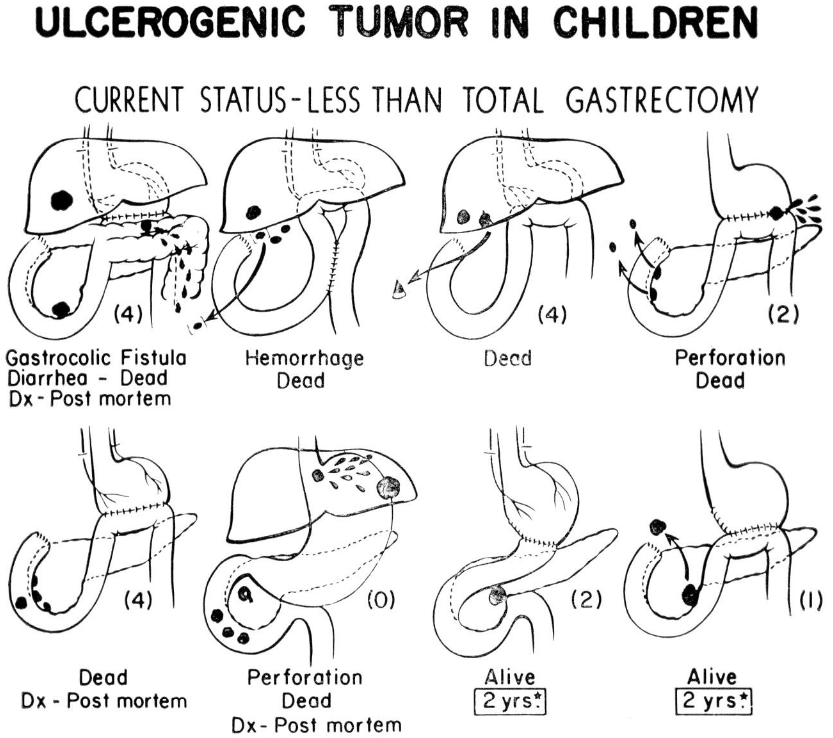

Figure 30. Long-time studies by Stuart Wilson *et al.*, showing a prolonged survival in childhood following total gastrectomy for an ulcerogenic tumor.

severe electrolyte imbalance will result unless there is cautious parenteral and oral fluid replacement of losses occurred by diarrhea or gastric aspiration. Considerable confirmatory diagnostic evidence can be obtained by a careful gastric analysis including an overnight aspiration which, not infrequently, will contain 2 L of gastric juice with a free acid content of 100 to 300 mEq/L. This is compared to a normal volume of 400 ml and an acid content of 13 mEq/L. It is important in carrying out the gastric analysis that the tube be placed at the most dependent portion of the stomach and its location verified by fluoroscopy. An output of 100 mEq/hr is not at all uncommon and should suggest, in the absence of pyloric obstruction, an extragastric cause for the marked hypersecretion. (Fig. 31) In addition, fixed acid output of more than 10

ULCEROGENIC TUMOR
Keys to Diagnosis (Lab)

Gastric analysis	
Massive hypersecretion	**100 ml/hr**
Fixed acid output	**> 10 mEq/hr**
Fixed acid concentration	**> 100 mEq**
Basal/stim. ratio	**0.6+**
Increased by calcium infusion	
Gastrin immunoassay	

Figure 31. Studies by gastric analysis supplemented by calcium infusion studies and simultaneous gastrin immunoassay studies should result in a high incidence of correct diagnosis.

mEq/hr and a fixed acid concentration of more than 100 mEq/L all tend to be confirmatory of the presence of an ulcerogenic tumor. Strong support has been given by many to the observation that the hypergastrinemia is stimulating the parietal cells to maximum output at all times, so that there is little change following the administration of histamine. Ruppert and others[465] have found that the ratio of basal acid concentration to maximal acid concentration (BAC/MAC) is selective for the ulcerogenic tumor if it is above 0.6.

Winship and Ellison[486] called attention to the variability of gastric secretion studies, such as the augmented histamine test and 12-hour overnight aspiration in a study of eight patients with peptic ulcers. Four of their patients had proven ulcerogenic syndrome, while in the other four, the diagnosis was suspected but not confirmed at operation. They emphasized that in seven of the eight patients, there were striking variations in the secretory patterns observed on repeated testing. Thus, caution is warranted in the interpretation of gastric secretory studies in any patient suspected to have an ulcerogenic tumor. Way, Goldman, and Dunphy[554] have likewise called attention to the variability of the gastric analysis findings in their series of 25 patients. In our judgment, this procedure is so time-consuming and the results so variable that it will undoubtedly be replaced by the gastrin immunoassay.

Upper gastrointestinal barium studies often lend significant proof to a suspected preoperative diagnosis of ulcerogenic tumor.

The tumors themselves are usually so small that indirect signs, such as organ displacement or invasion of the stomach and duodenal C-loop are rarely detected. However, the characteristic signs of marked hypersecretion—huge gastric mucosal folds combined with a large "shaggy" appearing duodenum with or without an ulcer—provide invaluable hints to the alert radiologist who is thoroughly familiar with the clinical history and laboratory results. To this end, many valuable papers have appeared in the literature. As experience has been gained more and more, the first clue to the diagnosis of an ulcerogenic tumor is provided by the upper gastrointestinal series.

Several years before the ulcerogenic tumor syndrome was described, Forty and Barrett, in 1952,[733] pointed out changes in the third part of the duodenum associated with islet cell tumors of the pancreas. These authors found out before the islet cell ulcerogenic syndrome was described that the relationship between peptic ulceration of the third part of the duodenum and islet cell tumors of the pancreas was found in 5 of the 14 patients examined —including the two in the original report.

In 1960, Wermer and associates called attention to upper gastrointestinal tract alterations by x-ray in adenomatosis of the endocrine glands.[82]

Missakian *et al*[323] reported in 1965 that roentgenograms of the small bowel did not demonstrate any characteristic changes except for findings consistent with malabsorption or deficiency state. They did not find any characteristic findings in the stomach; however, they did emphasize that when ulceration is located distal to the duodenum, with dilatation beyond the ulcerated region and flocculation of barium in the distal portion of the duodenum and proximal portion of the jejunum, there were significant findings suggesting the presence of an ulcerogenic tumor. Zboralske and Amberg,[559] on the other hand, found features in the small bowel that were characteristic in 16 of 17 patients with the ulcerogenic syndrome in their studies. These characteristics included megaduodenum, small bowel edema, increased intraluminal fluid, and frequent dilatation of the jejunum. They also observed that on occasion the ileum was dilated, and they observed abnormalities in the colon in two patients. Christoforidis and Nelson,[356] in 1966, studied 14 patients from our service who had the ulcerogenic syndrome. They emphasized that roentgenological examinations insured some important proof for early diagnosis. They pointed out that according to the world literature, there is a primary esophageal ulcer present in 1 per cent of the cases and emphasized that 3 of the 14 patients they had examined who had resection of approximately 90 per cent of the stomach later showed distal esophageal ulceration. There were 2 to 14 cases that had ulcer of the stomach, but they believe that the most significant finding was markedly hypertrophied mucosal folds (Fig. 32). This was so marked as to suggest a diagnosis of protein-losing gastropathy or even lymphoma. They called attention to the marked amounts of gastric fluid, even after fasting, and the lack of any organic obstruction. They found ulcers of the duodenum in 9 of 14 patients and emphasized that ulcers distal to the bulb should always raise suspicion of the ulcerogenic syndrome.

Postresection or marginal ulceration were described by Nelson and Christoforidis (Fig. 33) as tending to be deep, penetrating, and multiple. The ulcerations tended to be on the mesenteric border of the efferent loop rather than the usual marginal location.

Clemett and Park, in 1967,[411] reported a case in which selective

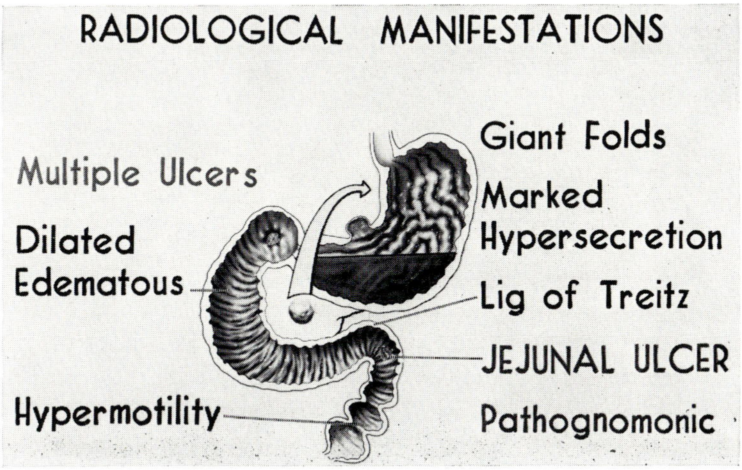

Figure 32. X-ray manifestations of the Zollinger-Ellison Syndrome. The diagnosis is often made by upper gastrointestinal examination.

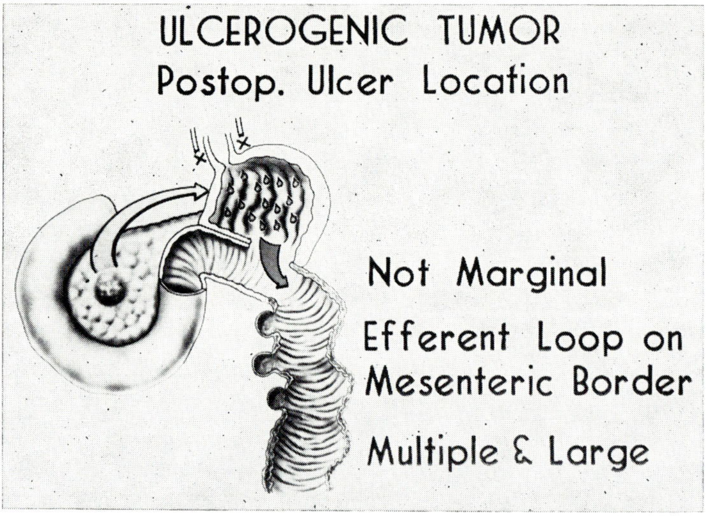

Figure 33. Nelson and Christoforidis have reported that the finding of multiple ulcers in the efferent loop rather than a marginal location suggests an ulcerogenic tumor as the etiology of a postoperative ulcer.

celiac arteriography showed a large area of hypervascularity in the body of the pancreas. A dense, irregular tumor stain persisted for several seconds. The selective superior mesenteric arteriogram was normal. A tumor was found involving the body of the pancreas, with evidence of local invasion at the time of operation. They called attention to the fact that non-beta islet cell tumors, cystic adenomas, and pancreatic sarcomas could and have been studied by angiography.

Alfidi and associates reported a case of ulcerogenic islet cell tumor and referred to three other patients reported in the literature.[562] Arteriography showed opacification suggesting the presence of an arteriovenous shunt at the capillary level, possibly in the mucosa. They emphasized the extremely early return of contrast media to the venous circulation in the case reported, which may be related to the large amount of gastrin produced by the pancreatic islet cell tumors. On the other hand, when defects are shown within the liver, support is given to the supposition that these patients already have metastasis. Selective arteriography of the pancreas has shown up islet cell tumors due to the increased venous blushing which outlines the lesions, even at times when they are rather small in size. However, our experience in this regard has been relatively limited and unfruitful. Arteriograms can be used in the search for metastatic nodules in the liver and to follow the progress of therapy, be it total gastrectomy or chemotherapy, when metastatic nodules have been found present at the time of operation (Fig. 34).

While scanning of the pancreas with selenium 75 may occasionally show up a defect in the pancreas, the decision for or against operative therapy in a patient suspected of an islet cell tumor is not dependent upon the results of the diagnostic procedure.

Following the discovery by Gregory that gastrin is the secretagogue present in ulcerogenic tumors, investigators were challenged to develop a diagnostic test which could measure this substance directly. Ghosh and Schild,[18] then Lai[273] (Fig. 35),

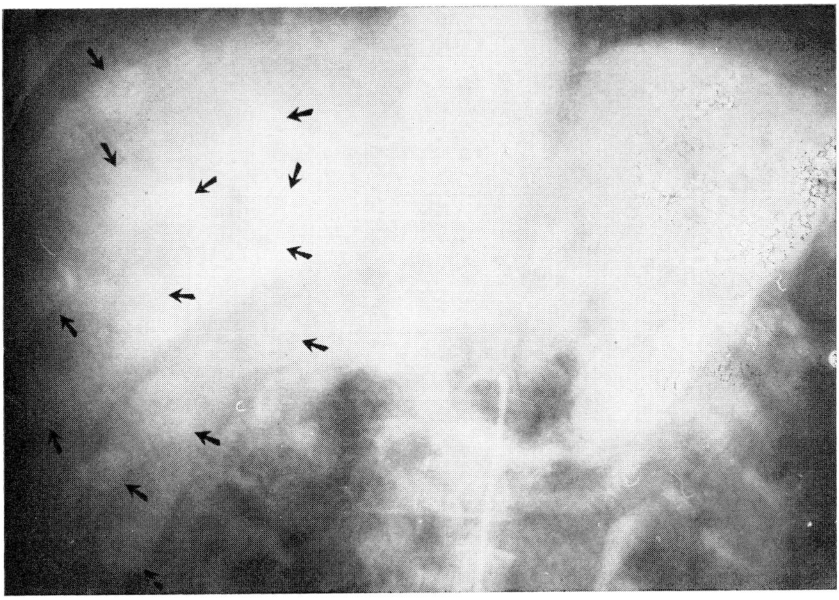

Figure 34. Aortogram showing multiple metastatic nodules in the liver one year after total gasterectomy.

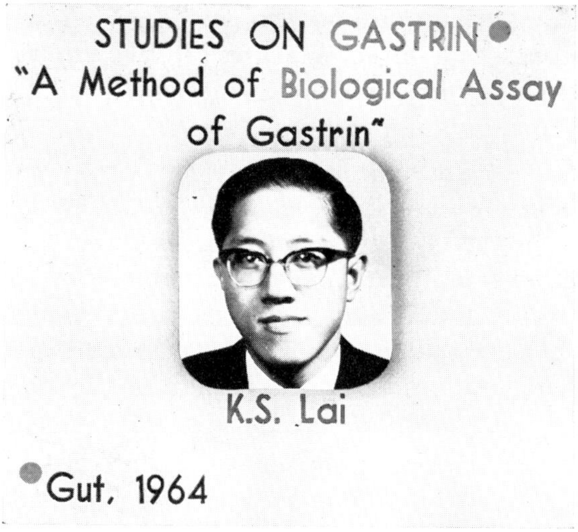

Figure 35. Dr. K. S. Lai, whose biological assay for gastrin proved to be a useful tool in diagnosis of gastrinemia.

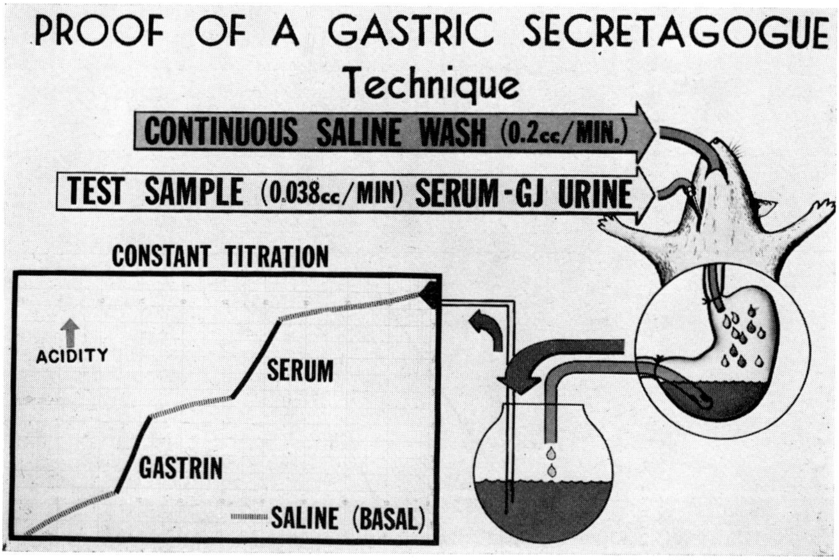

Figure 36. A schematic outline of the Lai bioassay which is a modification of Ghosh and Schild's technique.

emphasized the value of the isolated rat stomach as a means of studying the effect of gastric secretagogues, a technic which was adopted by Moore[453] and Thompson and Sircus[665] for the diagnosis of the ulcerogenic tumor syndrome (Fig. 36). Thompson and Sircus reported the value of the Lai preparation based on perfusion of the isolated rat stomach and the output of gastric acidity following the intravenous administration of serum, pH-adjusted gastric juice, or urine. Moore and his colleagues reported their experiences with this technic in 130 patients, 10 of whom had a positive response. Consistently positive results were obtained in all but one ulcerogenic tumor patient, who had variable responses. Wilson *et al*, in 1968[556] found evidence favoring a potent gastric secretagogue in only 10 of 15 patients, with proven ulcerogenic

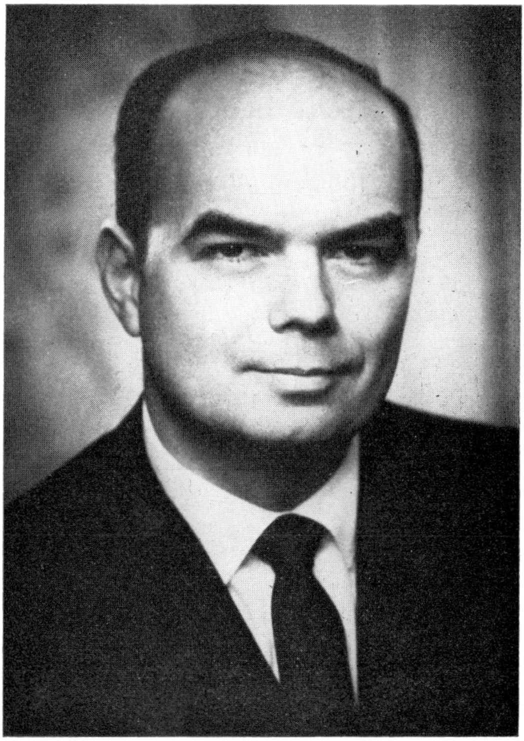

Figure 37. Dr. James E. McGuigan pioneered the development of the gastrin immunoassay in 1967.

tumors. The bioassay was negative in 21 control patients and in 22 patients with proven peptic ulcers. They emphasized that a negative bioassay did not necessarily rule out the presence of an ulcerogenic tumor, since there is a wide range of gastrin levels in such patients.

Bader, Bonfils, Lambling, and their associates[318,351,397] have made many notable contributions proving that there is a gastric secretagogue (which they call PSU-urinary secretagogue), in the urine of patients with ulcerogenic tumors. Wilken[616] and Thomson, Cleator, and Sircus[665] have both studied the factors affecting the bioassay of gastrin in anesthetized rats. Both groups concluded that the Lai bioassay is of diagnostic value and has practical advantages over other methods if the variables which affect the preparation can be held to a minimum.

In 1968, McGuigan (Fig. 37) reported the development of a sensitive radioimmunoassay technique for the measurement of gastrin concentrations in serum and plasma. He utilized this technic to quantitate the excessive amounts of gastrin in the serum of patients with the ulcerogenic syndrome and to document its presence in extracts of the non-beta islet cell tumor.[528]

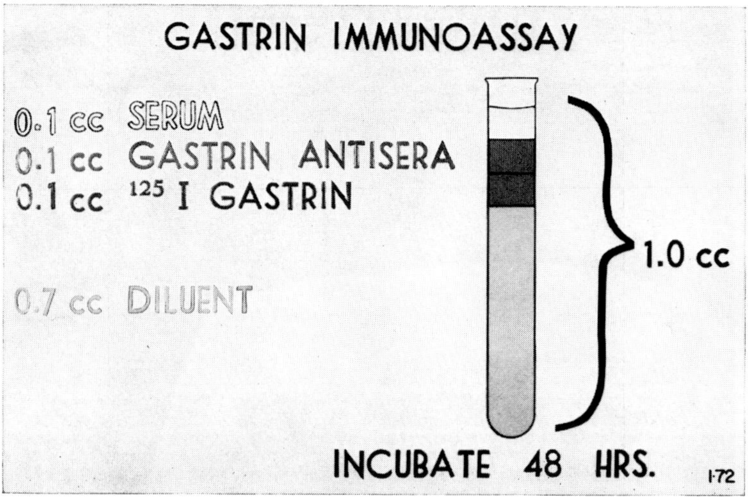

Figure 38. The four components in the gastrin immunoassay are incubated for 48 hours.

Several other groups of investigators have subsequently confirmed this monumental observation* (Figs. 38, 39, 40, 41). Concentrations of serum gastrin in normal fasting persons, reported by various authors, are in general agreement. Korman, Soveny, and Hansky found a mean fasting serum gastrin level of 32.1 ± 4.3 (SEM) pg/ml in 93 patients.[691] Yalow and Berson noted gastrin levels that were immeasurably low (< 75 pg) in nearly half of the 63 patients they examined.[704] McGuigan and Trudeau have reported a mean fasting serum gastrin concentration of $85 + 9.8$ pg/ml in 35 subjects without recognized gastrointestinal disease.[699]

However, reported gastrin levels in patients with duodenal ulcer disease are controversial. Hansky and Cain[691] and also Trudeau and McGuigan have found low to normal levels; others have reported variable levels (Walsh, Yalow, Berson) and Byrnes, Young, Chisholm, and Lazarus have reported high levels in this disease. Trudeau and McGuigan explain the low levels of serum gastrin in patients with duodenal ulcer on the basis of an inverse

* See references 590, 633, 650, 670, 676, 686, 691, 697, 704.

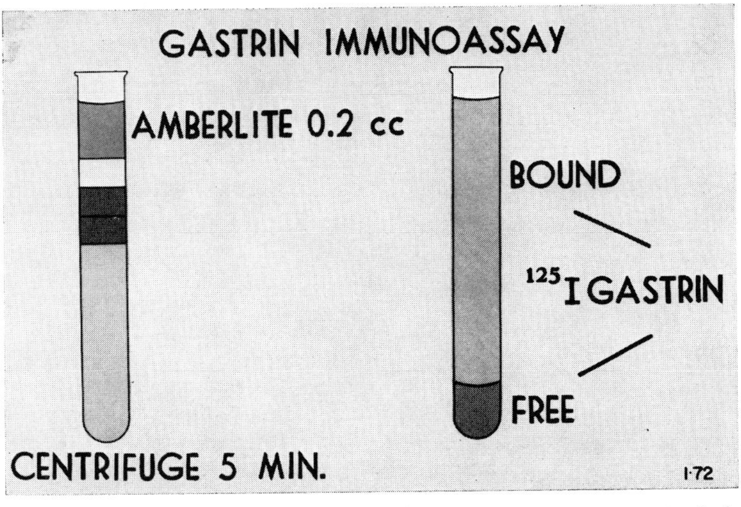

Figure 39. Amberlite is added and the components are mixed before centrifugation to separate the bound from the free gastrin.

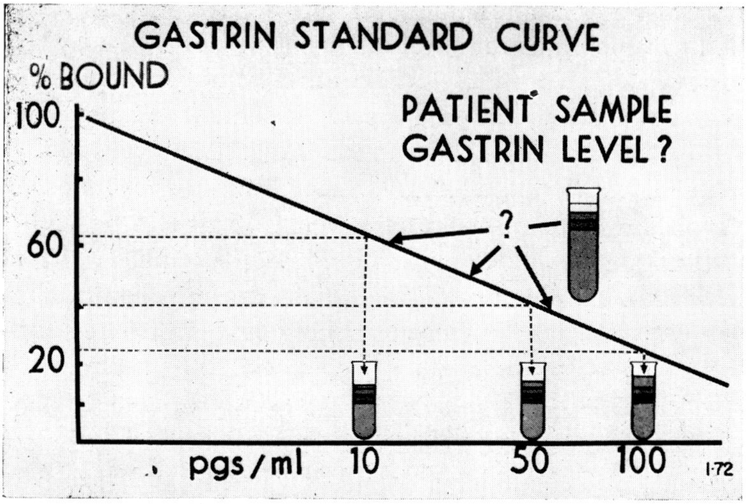

Figure 40. Gastrin levels determined by comparing per cent of bound gastrin in the patient's sample to a standard curve determined from known amounts of gastrin.

relation between fasting serum gastrin concentration and rates of gastric-hydrochloric acid secretion.[697]

Markedly elevated levels of serum gastrin in patients with pernicious anemia also support this concept. It has been suggested that because of the high intragastric pH in these patients, gastrin release is uninhibited and therefore serum gastrin levels are grossly elevated. This concept is supported by the observations of Yalow and Berson, who found that prompt and substantial reductions in elevated plasma-gastrin concentrations occurred in patients with pernicious anemia after ingestion of 0.1N hydrochloric acid.

GASTRIN IMMUNOASSAY *

	Picograms/Milliliter
Normal	0-100
Duodenal ulcer	100-300
Ulcerogenic syndrome	500-5000

*** OSU Levels**

Figure 41. Serum gastrin levels obtained in the surgery residents' laboratories using a modification of the Yalow and Berson technique.

Other physiologic studies have demonstrated increased serum levels of gastrin with increasing age, after eating, and also following the administration of calcium by mouth or intravenously.

The report by Trudeau and McGuigan that the infusion of calcium resulted in an increase in gastrin levels in a patient with ulcerogenic tumor suggested that this test might be valuable in the diagnosis of the borderline ulcerogenic tumor case. Passaro has reported the use of an intravenous calcium infusion (15 mg/kg body weight per 4 hrs) and has shown that in patients with the ulcerogenic syndrome, this produces a gastric acid secretion response at least 75 per cent of that seen after stimulation by histamine.[656] More recently, he has advocated the use of a smaller calcium dose (2 mg/kg) given intravenously as a bolus over a period of one minute, while measuring gastric acid secretion every 15 minutes for 1 hour. His studies indicate that the calcium load may be worthwhile as a screening test for an ulcerogenic tumor when gastrin immunoassay is not available.

Other studies by Sanzenbacher *et al.** have suggested that calcium infusion with concomitant serum gastrin determinations may be helpful in determining the progress of residual islet cell tumors or metastases following total gastrectomy. Since almost 70 per cent of the patients will have multicentric foci, including multiple adenomas of the pancreas, tumors within the duodenal wall, and metastases to adjacent lymph nodes and liver, the surgeon can never be sure he has removed all the tumor producing the potent gastric secretagogue. Measurement of the calcium-mediated serum gastrin may provide an effective means for evaluating these patients in the early and late postoperative period and may also offer a reliable method of determining if tumor growth is suppressed after total gastrectomy. The gastrin immunoassay yields quantitative results and as the test becomes more widely available should make the diagnosis of the ulcerogenic tumor more specific than possible from clinical and laboratory evidence available to the clinician in the past. Markedly elevated gastrin levels may well prove very useful to the surgeon in cases where

---

* Sanzenbacher, L. J., King, D. R. and Zollinger, R. M. Prognostic Implications of Calcium-Mediated Gastrin Levels in the Ulcerogenic Syndrome. Am. J. Surg. Vol. 125, Jan. 1973

he has been unable to find any evidence of tumor at the time of operation. While total gastrectomy has ordinarily not been recommended in the absence of documented tumor, the gastrin immunoassay could alter this position in that extremely high levels would prove very reassuring as an indication for total gastrectomy.

Passaro and colleagues[622,656] have recently emphasized the value of a calcium infusion as a potent stimulus for acid secretion in patients with an ulcerogenic tumor. They found in studying four patient with histologically proven non-beta islet cell tumors that the acid response to calcium infusion equalled by 70 per cent or exceeded the maximum acid response to Histalog® stimulus. On the other hand, the acid response to the calcium infusion in duodenal ulcer patients was only one-third that of the response to the Histalog. The authors suggested that calcium potentiated the response to gastrin and stimulated its release from the tumor. It is a test that can be used in screening for ulcerogenic tumors and may well prove to be a good indicator of functional activity of any lesions left behind. We have verified this response in several patients with ulcerogenic tumors and it should be a useful supplement in the absence of a gastrin immunoassay. The test is carried out after an overnight fast and aspiration, with discard of the 12-hour gastric aspiration. Following collection of a 15-minute basal secretion, an infusion of calcium gluconate (15 mg/kg body weight) is given for four hours, with gastric acid determinations every 30 minutes. Calcium gluconate, 2 mg/kg of body weight, may be used over a period of one hour as a short screening test.

SURGICAL TREATMENT OF THE ULCEROGENIC TUMOR SYNDROME

General Principles

Treatment of the ulcerogenic tumor entails two separate but intertwined considerations. Primary, but more lethal, are those related to the fulminating ulcer diathesis. Second are those caused by growth of the tumor itself. Faced with such a patient, the surgeon may choose one of two alternative courses of treatment: remove the primary source of gastrin by excision of the tumor, or remove its target or end-organ by total gastrectomy. *Success will be contingent upon removal of either all of the tumor or all of the acid-secreting surface.* Rare indeed is the patient with an ulcerogenic tumor who escapes operation; and indirect methods of therapy, such as massive doses of anticholinergics, chemotherapy, or irradiation, have, in general, been ineffective. The morbidity associated with ulcerogenic tumors is distressing and the mortality high; however, growth of the tumor and its metastases is slow and not at all incompatible with longevity. The real danger lies in their potent hormonal stimulation of gastric hypersecretion with all of its attendant complications. Treatment should therefore be designed to prevent the lethal effects of recurrent ulceration.

A few dramatic cures have accompanied local excision of a solitary pancreatic tumor or an aberrant adenoma within the wall of the duodenum or the gastric antrum. Unfortunately almost two thirds of the patients with multiple foci of tumor cells in the form of metastases or diffuse adenomatosis which are capable of producing the clinical syndrome if even a small rim of acid-secreting surface is left behind (Fig. 42). Likewise, total pancreatectomy affords no protection against recurrent ulceration if local or distant

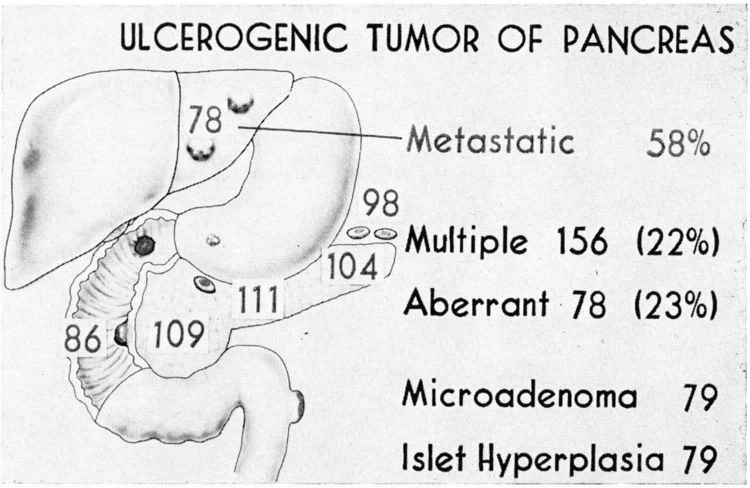

Figure 42. This drawing shows the multicentric potential location of gastrin producing tumors and metastases which make total gastrectomy the most effective form of controlling the ulcer diathesis.

metastases, microadenomata, or aberrant tumors are overlooked. Furthermore, there will be the daily need for specific and expensive replacement therapy.

Total gastrectomy after microscopic verification of the tumor or persistently high serum gastrin levels associated with marked gastric hypersecretion remains in our judgment the most beneficial procedure for the majority of patients with an ulcerogenic tumor of the pancreas. All potential for future ulcerogenesis is removed, even if tumor has knowingly or unknowingly been left behind. This radical procedure is also warranted in the presence of extensive hepatic metastases, even for an elderly patient, since it avoids the subsequent dangers of hemorrhage, perforation, peritonitis, and persistent ulcer-type pain. In general, patients who have undergone total gastrectomy for an ulcerogenic tumor experience far less difficulty in maintaining proper nutrition than when this same procedure is carried out for carcinoma. Finally, there is a growing body of evidence that total gastrectomy results in regression of any remaining tumor.

If it is possible for the surgeon to remove all of the ulcerogenic tumor by local excision, there is seldom anything to be gained by the addition of a radical gastric procedure. The combination of total gastrectomy and total pancreatectomy is indeed disastrous and one to be avoided.

Preoperative Preparation

The patients suspected of having an ulcerogenic tumor should be fully informed before surgery why it may be necessary to perform total gastrectomy together with splenectomy and partial resection of the pancreas. Considerable time is required to inform the family and to allay their fears when they learn that the entire stomach may be removed. Such informed consent must be obtained from any patient having surgery for recurrent ulceration following previous gastric resection for those with gigantic volumes of gastric secretion rich in hydrochloric acid or when there is evidence of hypercalcemia associated with hypersecretion and ulcer, and also in those relatively uncommon instances of gastrojejunocolic fistula. The surgeon must not be restricted in his approach at the time of surgery because the patient has not been well informed preoperatively.

It should be emphasized that the preoperative preparation of suspected ulcerogenic tumor patients must be energetic and carefully planned. Since the majority will have undergone one or many gastric operations, copies of the previous operative notes should be obtained as quickly as possible. The details of all previous operations, including the gastric analyses performed before or after them, are extremely important.

1. Was the surgeon specific that both vagus nerves had been divided? Was there microscopic evidence that both had been sectioned?
2. If vagotomy was not done, what was the extent of resection and the type of anastomosis?
3. Was there mention of considerable difficulty in freeing up the duodenum and closing the duodenal stump, suggesting a rim of retained antrum?
4. Did the surgeon pass his finger into the opened duodenum and palpate carefully for any irregularities which would suggest aberrant pancreas or one or more small islet cell tumors within the wall of the duodenum?
5. Was there evidence of an ulcer in the jejunum beyond the ligament of Treitz or a past history of a free perforation of such an ulcer?
6. After mobilization of the head of the pancreas by a Kocher maneuver, was there a thorough palpation of the pancreas from head to tail, including complete encirclement of the left half of the pancreas to permit palpation between the surgeon's thumb and index finger?
7. Was there a constant and copious output of gastric acid juice during the operation and/or the early postoperative period?
8. Did postoperative problems with gastric emptying lead to an enteroenterostomy as an emergency procedure?

The preoperative evaluation of patients suspected of having an ulcerogenic tumor is often closely related to their fluid and electrolyte balance, particularly if there has been a severe diarrhea or if large volumes of gastric juice have been aspirated each day.

Patients have been observed to lose ten pounds overnight because of excessive fluid losses. These patients should also have their weights monitored in the morning and in the evening, as a further check on their fluid needs. Furthermore, it may be necessary to administer unusually large amounts of electrolytes, particularly chloride and potassium, to bring the patients into balance. If dehydration or hypercalcemia have been a problem, then surgery should be delayed, if possible, until the serum levels of blood-urea-nitrogen and creatinine are within or nearly approach normal limits.

Those individuals who have had previous surgery and have evidence of a gastrojejunocolic fistula will, of course, require special consideration, including attempts at sterilization of the large bowel. On occasion, such patients will improve if they are hospitalized on a high caloric diet combined with a non-absorbable medication for sterilizing the colon.

The blood volume should preferably be measured and restored to normal levels before the operation.

Surgical Procedure

The type of definitive surgical procedure can only be determined after tumor has been verified by meticulous exploration of the entire pancreas, the duodenum, and the gastric antrum. Regional lymph nodes and the liver are carefully examined for evidence of metastases.

The patient should be placed on the operating table nearest the side of the surgeon. Since the operation may be a rather prolonged one, it is essential that adequate provisions have been made for fluid, electrolyte, and blood replacement during the procedure. In a patient with no previous operative treatment, a midline incision is made from the xyphoid to the umbilicus for the preliminary exploration. All too many of these patients have one or more scars on the upper abdomen from previous surgery, and considerable time may be required to evaluate which incision should be reopened to ensure adequate exposure with a minimum chance of a postoperative hernia. Usually the one nearest the midline is preferred.

Since a thorough exploration of the pancreas, stomach, duodenum, and liver will be required, liberal exposure is advisable which extends well below the left side of the umbilicus and well up over the xyphoid process. The zyphoid process is usually removed to ensure better exposure, particularly if it is quite prominent and if total gastrectomy is to be performed.

Great care should be taken in opening the peritoneal cavity, particularly in patients having had previous surgery, because of the frequent presence of penetration of a stomal ulceration up against the anterior parietes.

Indirect evidence that a tumor is present will become apparent as soon as the peritoneal cavity is opened. This includes marked vascularity of the stomach and great thickness of the mucosa, which is definitely apparent on palpation. The duodenum is definitely enlarged, and further deformity might be present, often in the second or third portion of the duodenum. When the patient has had previous surgery, there may be findings which resemble a low-grade inflammatory process throughout the entire abdomen, with many filmy adhesions between the loops of small intestine.

Usually the first and second portions of the duodenum are first freed up by a Kocher maneuver which permits inspection of the anterior and posterior walls and direct palpation of the head of the pancreas and the deeper areas around the portal vein. The wall of the duodenum, particularly along the mesenteric border, is carefully palpated for tumor nodules arising from aberrant pancreas. The surgeon may also split the pylorus and explore the lument of the first and second portions of the duodenum in an effort to discover intramural adenomata. As a next step, the omentum is reflected upward and the upper jejunum surveyed for some distance because of the relatively high incidence of primary jejunal ulcerations occurring beyond the ligament of Treitz. When this is the initial operation on the upper gastrointestinal tract, the first step is not only to verify the presence of an ulcer but also to weigh the evidence for or against an ulcerogenic tumor either within or apparent on the surface of the pancreas, or metastastic to the regional lymph nodes and liver.

After verifying the amount of obvious pathology, the greater omentum is separated from the hepatic flexure to the splenic flexure of the colon in order to attain complete exposure of the pancreas from one end to the other. The greater omentum is reflected upward, and downward traction is maintained on the transverse colon as the omentum is separated by sharp dissection and the lesser sac entered. After the omentum has been completely dissected off the colon and all bleeding points have been ligated, the stomach is retracted upward and the entire body and tail of the pancreas is inspected for evidence of a tumor. Since these tumors are usually quite small, they may not be apparent by gross inspection or palpation. In this case, the surgeon must mobilize the body and tail of the pancreas for direct palpation. In our judgment, it is doubtful if a completely satisfactory exploration of the body and tail of the pancreas can be accomplished without complete mobilization of the spleen and body and tail of the pancreas toward the midline. To accomplish this, the splenic flexure is detached, the splenocolic ligament divided, and the entire transverse colon, including the splenic flexure, is retracted downward. It is advisable to divide the short gastrosplenic vessels and the splenorenal ligament, as well as the peritoneum along the inferior surface of the pancreas, in order that the spleen and tail of the pancreas can be gently mobilized toward the midline. Blunt finger dissection easily develops a cleavage plane which permits freeing up of the posterior aspect of the pancreas. Actually, the index finger can be introduced up and around the splenic vessels running along the superior margin of the pancreas to permit more direct palpation of any suspicious areas within the left half of the pancreas, without mobilizing the spleen. Great care must be taken to avoid injuring the mesenteric vein as it comes up to join the splenic vein just behind the body of the pancreas. Such mobilization enables the surgeon to palpate for any unusual thickness or discreet nodule from almost the region of the portal vein to the tip of the pancreas. Furthermore, it permits direct visualization of the posterior wall of the body and tail of the pancreas. Any enlarged lymph nodes or small nodules over the pancreas should be excised and sent to the pathologist for frozen section examination.

When complete mobilization fails to disclose tumor by thorough palpation of the head, body and tail of the pancreas, including the region of the portal vein, it may be advisable to proceed with a "blind" resection of the left half of the pancreas in a search for small tumors or adenomatosis. The surgeon should take the position, however, that it is essential to have microscopic evidence of an islet cell tumor before proceeding with total gastrectomy at the time of the initial operation. If such is not gained, the surgeon can go ahead with his favorite gastric resection or pyloroplasty, realizing that a second operation might become mandatory in a distressingly short period of time. High serum gastric levels in the presence of high acid values lend strong support for total gastrectomy, even in the absence of microscopic proof of tumor.

If there is obvious evidence of a tumor on the left side of the pancreas, the surgeon may either partially enucleate it for microscopic examination, or the entire left side of the pancreas together with the spleen can be resected. The splenic artery and vein are doubly ligated and the tail of the pancreas closed with interrupted mattress sutures of silk. The resected pancreas should be immediately sectioned by the surgeon in order that he may search for evidence of a suspicious nodule or small adenoma, as indicated by small, white nodules within the substance of the gland. When a non-beta islet cell tumor is found and substantiated microscopically, most authors have invariably recommended that total gastrectomy be carried out. The tendency to resort to vagotomy, antrectomy, and other lesser procedures in the presence of an ulcerogenic tumor, particularly when they are multiple, is only inviting disaster.

One of the greatest difficulties encountered by the surgeon is his inability to prove the presence of an ulcerogenic non-beta islet cell tumor of the pancreas, even in the face of overwhelming clinical and laboratory evidence pointing to it. This can be a most challenging search, particularly in patients having had two or three previous gastric operations, with areas of marked inflammatory reaction and dense adhesions between the anterior surface of the pancreas and adjacent structures. Preoperative evidence of serially high serum gastrin levels by immunoassay may eventually make the surgeon's decision a much easier one. Until that time, the surgeon should first eliminate the many iatrogenic causes of recurrent ulceration. It is advisable to make certain that all vagus nerves have been divided, particularly the posterior one, regardless of the number of previous operations. The surgeon must also evaluate the closure of the duodenal stump, since an overlooked small rim of antrum following a Billroth II procedure can bring about a clinical syndrome which closely mimics that of the ulcerogenic tumor. Finally, the small bowel should be carefully evaluated for an enteroenterostomy or long-loop gastrojejunal anastomosis which might predispose the patient to recurrent ulcerations.

When an ulcerogenic tumor has been found and proven microscopically at either a primary or subsequent operation, the decision in favor of total gastrectomy is not at all difficult. After double ligation of the right gastric and the right gastroepiploic vessels, the duodenum is divided and the lumen explored with the index finger. The duodenal stump is then closed with a layer of interrupted 0000 silk, with an inversion layer of interrupted 00 silk mattress sutures. Since the omentum has already been freed from the colon, the stomach is retracted upward to expose the left gastric vessels. The left gastric artery is then doubly ligated. As a matter of fact, we have ligated the left gastric artery, with or without subtotal gastrectomy, in an effort to control massive gastric hypersecretion, even when an ulcerogenic tumor was not found and it was not believed advisable to proceed with total gastrectomy. This technical approach should also make subsequent removal of the remaining gastric pouch easier should such become necessary. The uppermost portion of the gastrohepatic ligament is likewise divided and transfixed on both sides with 00 silk. The spleen has usually been separated from the stomach as part of the mobilization of the spleen and tail of the pancreas for complete exploration of the pancreas.

Exposure of the lower end of the esophagus should be achieved carefully in order to avoid fraying of the nonperitonealized muscular esophageal wall. Since many of these patients have had previous vagotomy, there tend to be very dense adhesions between the superior surface of the left lobe of the liver and the overlying diaphragm. Sharp dissection is required to avoid tearing the capsule of the liver with resultant troublesome bleeding. Likewise, the undersurface of the left lobe of the liver is likely to be intimately attached to the underlying stomach in the region of the esophagogastric junction. It is important that the left lobe of the liver be freed up and mobilized toward the midline to ensure adequate exposure of the esophagogastric junction. As the mobilized left lobe is brought toward the midline, it is covered with a moist gauze pad which is held in position with a large S-retractor. The gastrohepatic ligament is then divided, and the thickened uppermost portion, which contains a branch of the inferior phrenic artery, is clamped and ligated. This ensures more direct exposure of the region posterior to the esophagus where the more commonly overlooked right vagus nerve is located.

The secondary exposure of the esophageal-gastric junction is not as easy as the initial operation, and for this reason the peritoneum is carefully incised up over the esophagus after identification of its location by palpation of the underlying nasogastric tube. Since the usual cleavage planes tend to be obliterated by scar tissue attachments, less fraying of the muscular wall will result if blunt dissection is carried out from above downward, rather than by the usual blind, left-to-right finger dissection. It is important to maintain the usual integrity of the muscular wall of the esophagus for the subsequent anastomosis when total gastrectomy is necessary.

After resection of both vagus nerves, the esophagus generally comes down at least 5 to 6 cm. into the abdominal cavity; however, it will tend to retract into the mediastinum when divided from the stomach unless it has been anchored at four points to the crus of the diaphragm with interrupted silk sutures (Fig. 43). Care should be taken to avoid penetrating the lumen of the esophagus during this maneuver. The esophageal wall at the point of division can be given further substance by placing a series of interrupted, encircling horizontal sutures of 0000 silk (Fig. 44). Such fixation prevents fraying of the muscles and tends to afford a firm cuff for the anastomosis. These sutures have not resulted in compromise of the blood supply to the anastomosis. Placement of median and lateral angle sutures will help to maintain proper orientation and prevent rotation of the esophagus as the anastomosis is carried out.

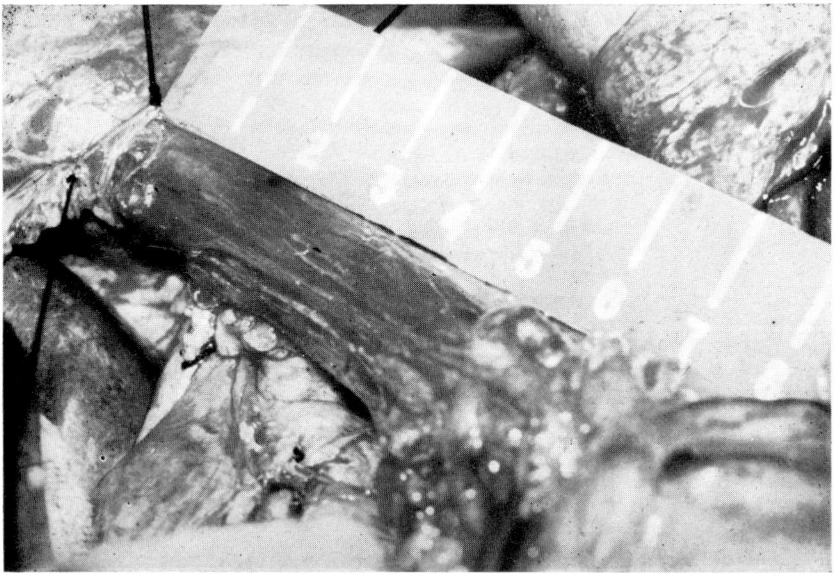

Figure 43. Following the division of the vagus nerve, the esophagus is elongated into the duodenum. The esophagus is fixed with several silk sutures to the hiatus to prevent retraction of the esophagus following division of the esophageal gastric junction.

A variety of postgastrectomy reconstructions have been recommended (Fig. 45). The Roux-en-Y and enteroenterostomy are probably the most common, however, some surgeons prefer construction of a Lawrence pouch or an interposition utilizing either the Longmire-Beal or the Poth technics. In general, the Roux-en-Y is a satisfactory anastomosis when performed end-to-side to the jejunum with the end of the jejunum directed most commonly to the left side. The blood supply to the upper jejunum must be evaluated repeatedly to determine the ideal point for its division prior to mobilizing either the free or the prolonged end of the jejunum. As previously mentioned, the tendency for increased vascularity of the intestine combined with the added thickness and inflammatory reaction in the mesentery makes the mobilization more difficult than in the usual ulcer patient. An opening is made in the mesocolon to the left of the middle colic vessels and through this, the loop of jejunum is tested for the feasibility

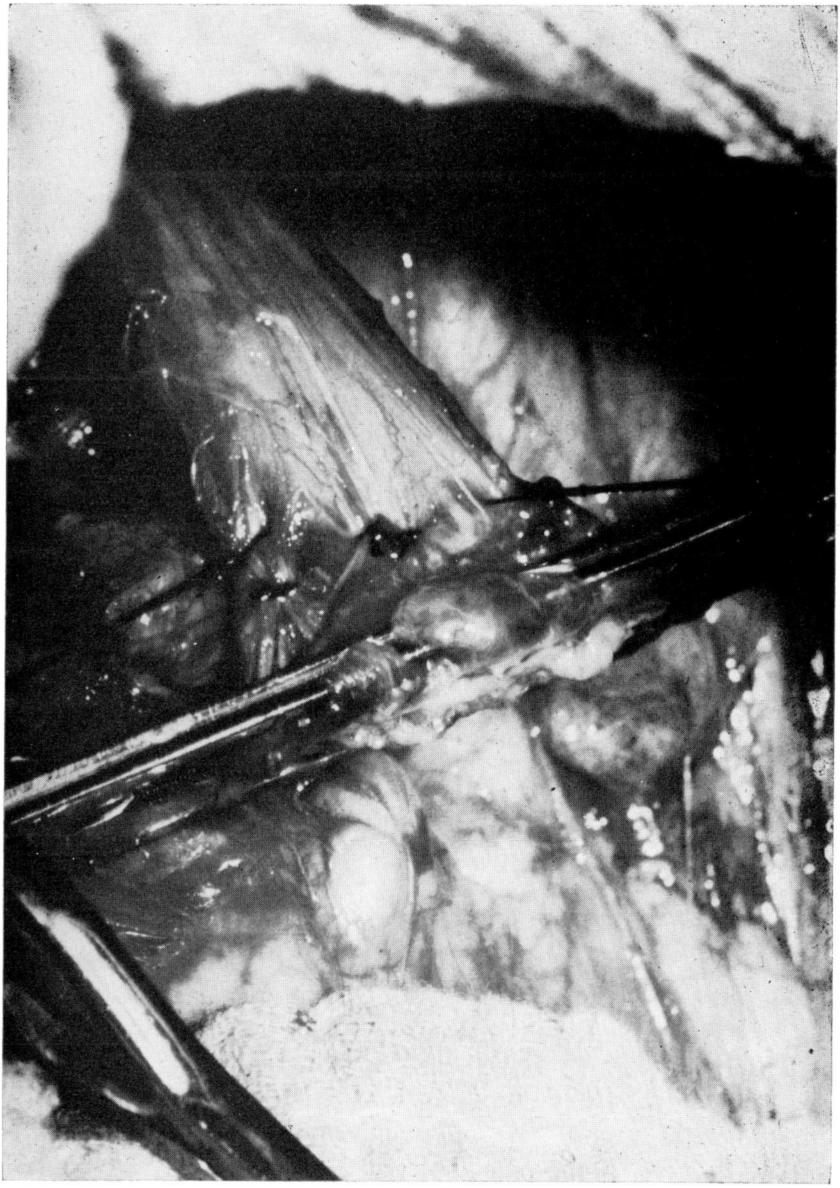

Figure 44. The esophagus is encircled with interrupted 0000 silk sutures to control bleeding and give a firm margin to the esophagus for the subsequent anastomosis to the jejunum.

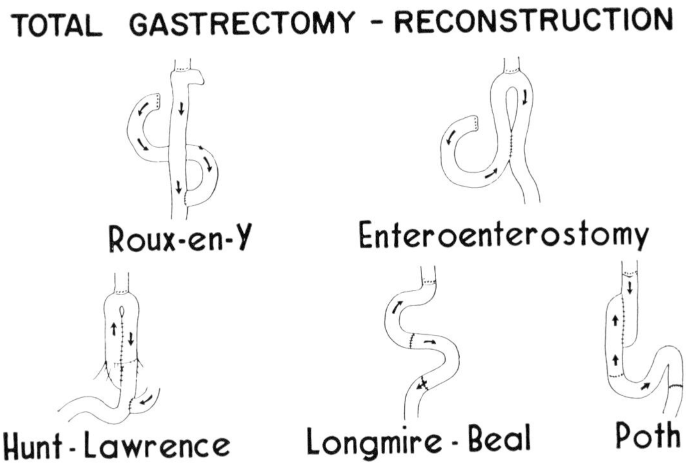

Figure 45. A variety of substitute reconstructions follow total gastrectomies. The senior author prefers the Roux-en-Y procedure, while others prefer interpositions in the hope of improving long-term nutrition.

of easily reaching up, without tension, to the base of the diaphragm in the region of the esophagus. Once a sufficient length of upper jejunum has been determined, the blood supply is palpated in the mesentery to assist in properly ligating only those blood vessels which are absolutely required for mobilization of the arm of the jejunum. The end of the jejunum is next closed with two layers of silk unless it is to be utilized as an interposition or to form some type of pouch. In order to accurately mark where the opening in the jejunum is to be made, it is often helpful to place traction sutures within a few centimeters of the closed end of the jejunum. This will outline the length of the subsequent incision in the bowel wall preparatory to the esophageal anastomosis. Next the jejunum is anchored to the diaphragm with a few interrupted sutures of 00 silk placed posterior to the esophagus. These sutures should be placed near the margins of the mesentery and as far away as possible from the proposed site of anastomosis in order to provide sufficient room for the two-layer closure which will follow.

An opening is next made between the traction sutures while they are held under traction to assure a lumen equivalent to that of the esophagus. The mucosa of the jejunum and esophagus are approximated with interrupted 0000 silk sutures. The stomach tube is then advanced down the arm of the jejunum, after which the anterior and lateral walls of the anastomosis are completed, utilizing inverted 0000 silk Connell sutures. A second, anterior layer of interrupted 00 silk sutures between the muscle layers and the jejunum is carried out and then the anterior wall and angles of the jejunum are once again anchored to the diaphragm to remove all tension from the completed three-layer suture line.

The transected end of the jejunum beyond the ligament of Treitz is now anchored to the base of the ascending limb with two layers of silk. It is important to close carefully any extra opening which may have been made in the mesocolon and also anchor the edges of the mesocolon to the jejunum to prevent any possible rotation of the mobilized arm of jejunum. Any openings below the "jejunal anastomosis" should be closed with interrupted sutures, with care taken to avoid injury to the blood vessels within the mesentery. Finally, the Levin tube is directed well down into the jejunum beyond the most distal anastomosis. Prior to closure of the wound, the adequacy of the blood supply to all portions of the mobilized jejunum should be verified once again and any abnormal openings about the mesentery double checked and closed with interrupted sutures. Drainage does not appear to be necessary unless a portion of the pancreas has been resected. Under these circumstances, adequate drainage of the left upper quadrant is instituted and directed toward the divided end of the pancreas. Some authors, on the other hand, prefer a sump type of drainage. A small polyethylene tube can be anchored in the end of the small pancreatic duct with fine catgut and brought out through a stab wound to insure free drainage of pancreatic juice during the early postoperative period.

It should be emphasized, at this point, that every surgeon has his own preference for establishing gastrointestinal continuity after total gastrectomy, and the foregoing discussion is in no way intended to emphasize the merits of one over another.

Postoperative Management

Routine and immediate postoperative care will vary with the individual surgeon; however, it is wise to develop a policy for the prolonged care of these patients. Slowly but surely, they should be started on six small feedings a day and be taught to keep track of their weight rather frequently. Vitamin B-12 injections should be given at least once a month and additional vitamin supplementation maintained as needed. As a general principle, it would seem beneficial to the patients to be readmitted within three months for restudy of their dietary habits and to check on the patency of the esophagojejunal anastomosis. At times, gentle dilatation of the anastomosis may relieve the patients of many of their symptoms and markedly increase their caloric intake. It may be hard for the patient and his family to realize that he can gradually return to a non-restricted diet, which is usually the case in a relatively short period of time. Blood sugar levels should be determined from time to time, searching for diabetes, particularly if a large segment of the pancreas has been removed. Serum gastrin levels should be determined every six months both before and after the infusion of calcium gluconate as a means of checking on the functional activity of any metastases which have been left behind and also to determine if the levels are subsiding in response to removal of the target organ.

The Effects of Total Gastrectomy on Tumor Regression

The finding of metastases in a lymph node adjacent to the pancreas in one of the original two patients reported in 1955, who has remained well for over 17 years, has stimulated considerable thought as to why metastases did not spread with a fatal result. It is now generally accepted that it is possible for a patient to have multiple metastases to the liver, yet live for many years without difficulty, while others seem to progress in the usual fashion. As far as can be determined, there is no particular cell type or location and extent of the metastases which can be used to predict the subsequent growth trend of the metastases.

Friesen, in particular, has been emphatic in pointing out the occasional spontaneous regression of the syndrome, and he refers to the patient reported by Melnyck, Krippaehne, and Dunphy.[322] Friesen carried out observations on serum gastrin levels in 33 patients, 19 without and 14 with the Zollinger-Ellison syndrome.[633]

There were six patients who had had a total gastrectomy with evidence of metastatic ulcerogenic tumor present. The remaining eight patients, with the syndrome included three treated by subtotal gastrectomy, two without proof of metastatic disease, two who had not had definite surgery, and one who had islet hyperplasia only. After this study, Friesen concluded that it is reasonable to recommend total gastrectomy for those who clearly meet the diagnostic criteria of the Zollinger-Ellison syndrome, with histological evidence of islet cell and/or metastasizing tumor which are elaborating a single hormone and evidence that gastrin levels in the serum are elevated. In 1967,[419] he had studied six patients with the syndrome, with special reference to the relationship of the clinical course of the disease with the treatment given. All of these patients had metastatic non-beta islet cell carcinoma, except one, who had diffuse islet cell hyperplasia. He pointed out that three of these patients treated by subtotal gastrectomy died, with evidence of fulminating ulcer complications and progressive metastases of carcinoma. He emphasized that the three patients in whom total gastrectomy was done were free of symptoms and had no evidence of islet cell tumor; two of these had metastatic islet cell carcinoma when a second-look operation was carried out four and five years after total gastrectomy. From these observations and the known slow growth of the metastases reported in the literature he raised the question of whether or not removal of the entire stomach influences the growth of pancreatic islet cells and, in short, tends to control the metastases.

Prognosis

The prognosis for the future of the patient having an ulcerogenic tumor is difficult to assess because the tumor tends to grow slowly despite the evidence at the time of surgery of gross metastases to adjacent lymph nodes and to the liver. Our original patient operated on in November, 1954, remains in good health and is the mother of two children; she has had a cholecystectomy, splenectomy and left-sided pancreatectomy, and a panhysterectomy in the intervening years. (Fig. 46, 47) Her only medication consists of B-12 at least once a month. Her weight has been

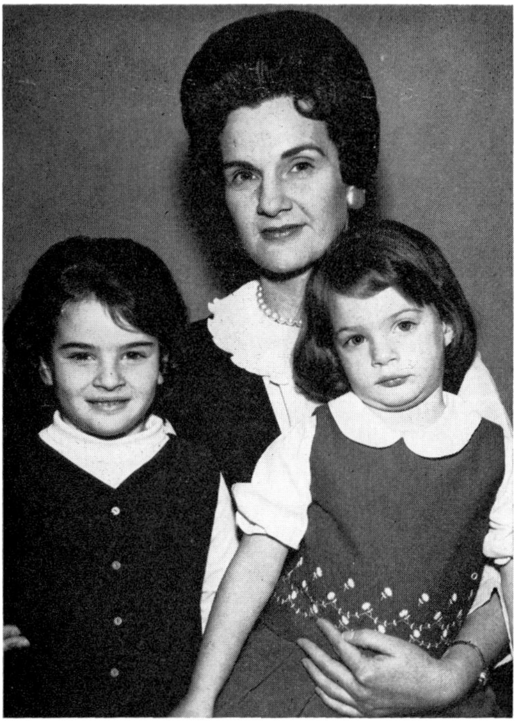

Figure 46. Photograph of one of the original two patients with ulcerogenic tumor who has had two children, 8 and 10 years following total gastrectomy.

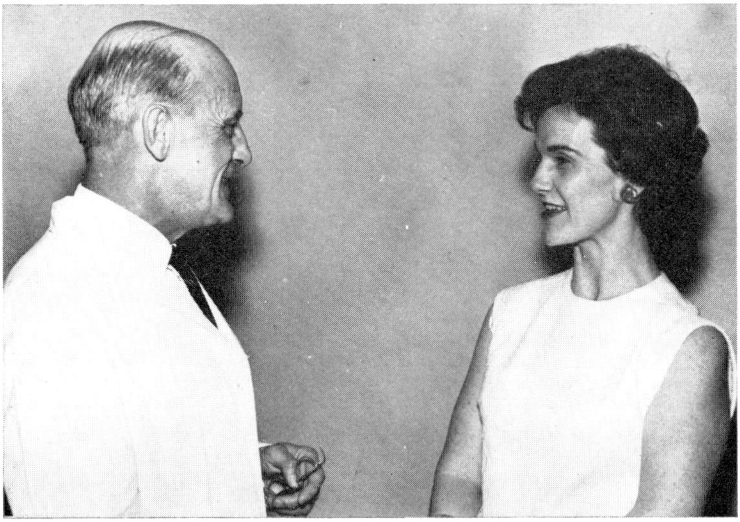

Figure 47. The distinguished physiologist Dr. R. A. Gregory, interviewing the first ulcerogenic tumor patient, Columbus, Ohio, in 1966.

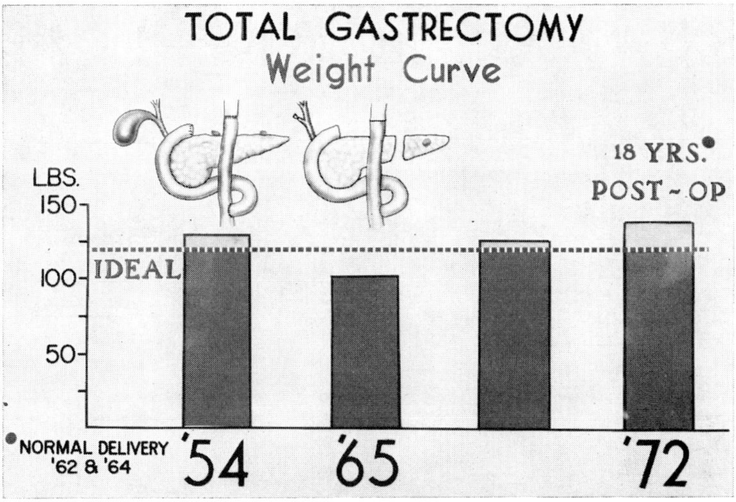

Figure 48. The weight curve following total gastrectomy remained surprisingly good in patients having an ulcerogenic tumor following total gastrectomy regardless of the type of esophageal jejunal reconstruction.

sustained at about 147 pounds, which is more than she wishes to weigh (Fig. 48). She has no limitations whatsoever insofar as diet is concerned. At the time of cholecystectomy, ten years after the original operation, when metastases to the local lymph nodes had been found, the left side of the pancreas was resected with the finding of a small benign microadenoma within the pancreas but no evidence of malignancy (Fig. 49).

It has been suggested, particularly by Friesen (Fig. 50), that removal of the target organ, namely the stomach, by total gastrectomy may inhibit the growth of the metastases (Fig. 51). However, on at least three occasions, patients have been seen who failed to recover and went progressively down-hill in the presence of solid, hard, sizeable metastases to the lymph nodes about the celiac axis and extensive metastases to the liver. However, it is certainly true that the chances of a prolonged survival in the presence of lymph node metastases is far different, as indicated from experience gained from the literature, than that expected from other types of malignant tumors. Whether or not this is the result of behavior of certain endocrine tumors or

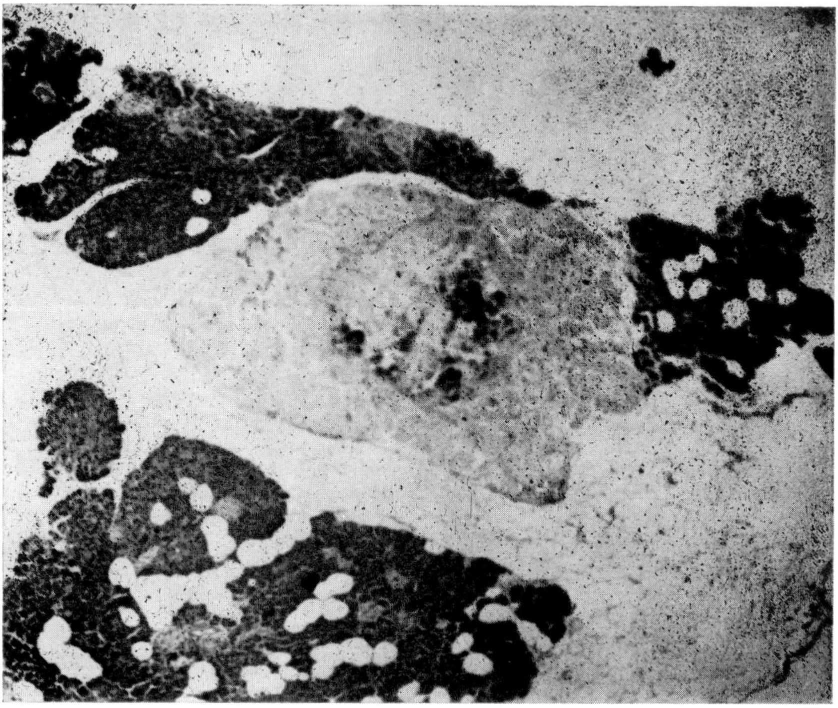

Figure 49. A small adenoma found in the left half of the pancreas when we operated on the original patient ten years after total gastrectomy. The surgical procedure was performed for treatment of cholecystitis and cholelithiasis.

carcinoid-like tumors cannot be determined at this time. Certainly the growth trend of the metastases will be more accurately evaluated in the future, when a worldwide availability of gastrin immunoassay to determine the trend of the hypogastrinemia is available following the total gastrectomy. Friesen has referred to the gastropituitary axis in which gastrin stimulates hydrochloric acid.[633] Hydrochloric acid, in turn, inhibits antral secretion. The antral inhibition stimulates the pituitary and the pituitary gastrotrophic hormone stimulates the production of gastrin, but this does not take place in the complete absence of the stomach. Support to this concept comes from the observation by Stadil *et al.* in their observation on a patient with a proven ulcerogenic tumor

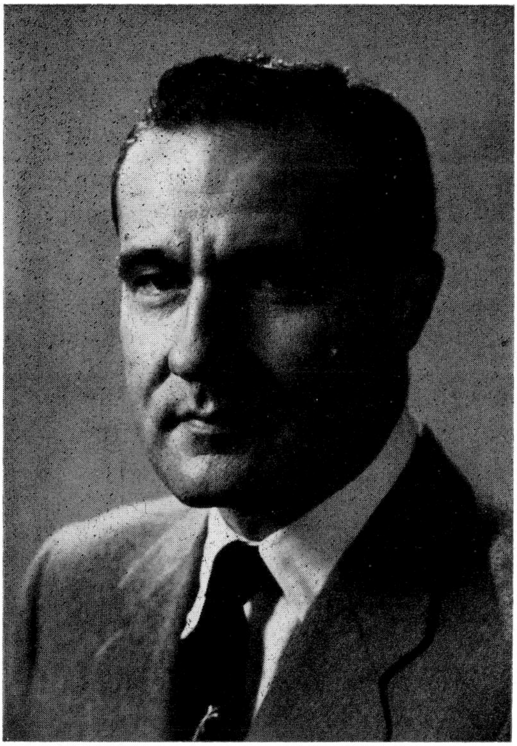

Figure 50. Dr. Stanley Friesen, Professor of Surgery, The University of Kansas, who has advocated the principle of regression of the metastases following total gastrectomy.

during the continued aspiration of gastric juice and the regular sampling of the peripheral venous blood with determination of the serum gastrin concentrations by radioimmunoassay.[704] They reported "the serum gastrin fell acutely within 10 minutes of the start of the aspiration and a basal level was reached after one hour. From 60 minutes after the start of aspiration secretin was given as a continuous intravenous infusion of 1 I.U. per kilogram per hour. This did not influence the level of gastrin in the serum." They carried out a second experiment where the serum gastrin concentrations were determined over a period of two hours with subsequent reinstillation of 200 cc of gastric juice. In their previous experiment, the concentration of gastrin decreased about 700 $\mu\mu$g/ml during aspiration (Fig. 52). However, reinstillation

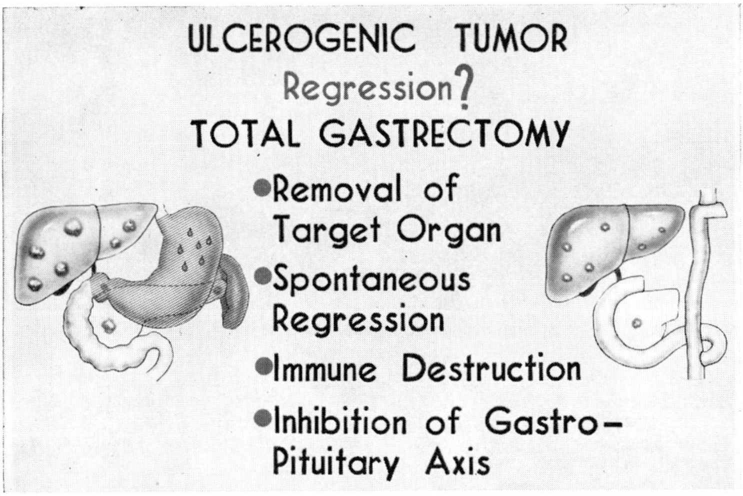

Figure 51. Some of the principles advocated in the proposal that removal of the stomach or, "target organ" results in regression of ulcerogenic tumor.

caused a steep increase of gastrin in serum within 10 minutes and a peak of 1,700 $\mu\mu$g was reached in about 1 hour. These observations were made in a young male patient with the ulcerogenic

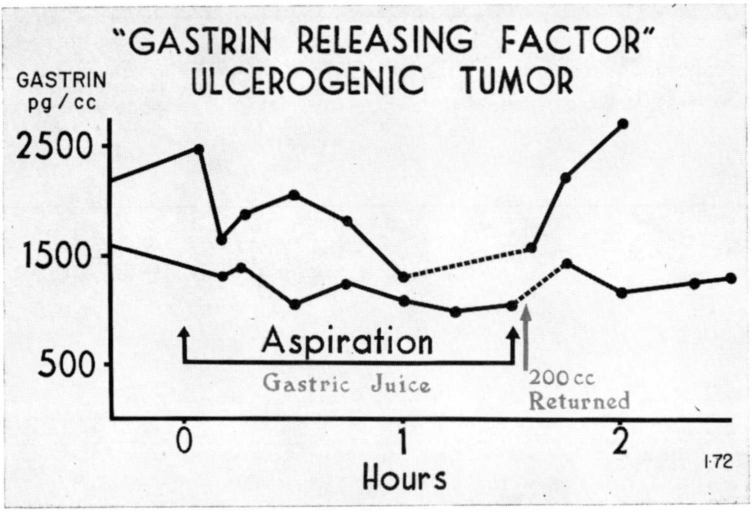

Figure 52. Serum gastrin levels tend to decline as gastric juice is aspirated from a patient with an ulcerogenic tumor and increase when the gastric juice is returned.

syndrome. Furthermore, they found that the serum gastrin concentration in the venous blood to the antrum was slightly lower, 300 $\mu\mu$g/ml, than in simultaneously drawn peripheral venous blood, 4100 $\mu\mu$g/ml.

They concluded that the decrease in the serum gastrin levels during aspiration of the gastric juice suggests an indirect effect of gastric juice on the gastrin-producing tumor. The authors suggest that their observations support the hypothesis of Friesen that the activities of the metastases are influenced by the acid-secreting mucosa of the stomach.

Following total gastrectomy, the calcium infusion test of Passaro may be used to monitor the gastrin-producing potential of any remaining tumor or metastasis. Observations on a series of patients 5 years after total gastrectomy following the infusion of 15 mg of calcium gluconate per kilogram of body weight showed no increase in the basal gastrin level in some patients, with elevated levels in others, especially after the administration of the calcium infusion test. The relatively normal fasting gastrin levels may be misleading, since several patients two and three years after total gastrectomy had a definite elevation of the serum gastrin levels over the fasting levels following the calcium infusion. This latter finding supports the persistence of active gastrin-producing metastases (Figs. 53, 54).

PATHOLOGY OF THE ULCEROGENIC AND DIARRHEOGENIC ISLET CELL TUMORS

Tumors of the pancreas have long challenged the pathologist because their identification by frozen section can be most difficult and the cell of origin of a particular tumor often defies identification. Many of the islet cell tumors can not be differentiated from carcinoid tumors, regardless of their hormonal activity. Ackey and Knopp[675] related that beta cells which produce insulin make up 75 per cent of the cellular elements that compose the one million or more islets of the pancreas. Approximately 20 per cent of the remainder were alpha cells which produce glucagon. The remaining 5 per cent of the cells have not been so universally agreed upon, but they are commonly referred to as delta cells.

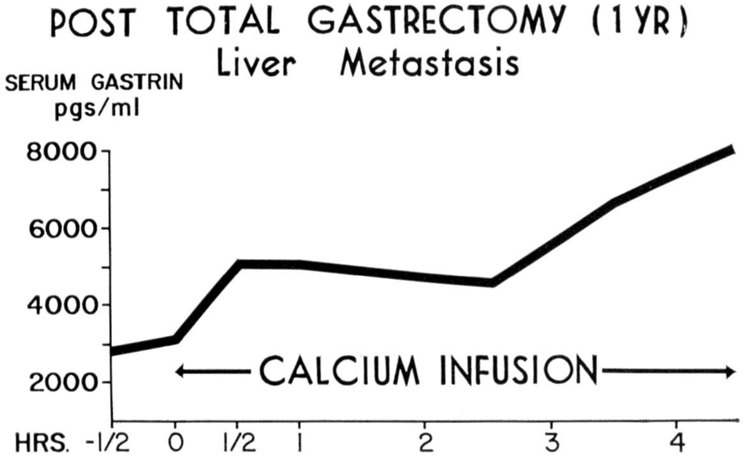

Figure 53. Calcium infusion study one year after total gastrectomy and 2-½ years after extensive hepatic metastases were demonstrated by arteriogram.

These later cells of debatable status have often been assigned the source of excessive gastrin in patients with the ulcerogenic islet cell syndrome, while the identification of the gastrin producing cell in the ulcerogenic islet cell tumor remains a problem. The

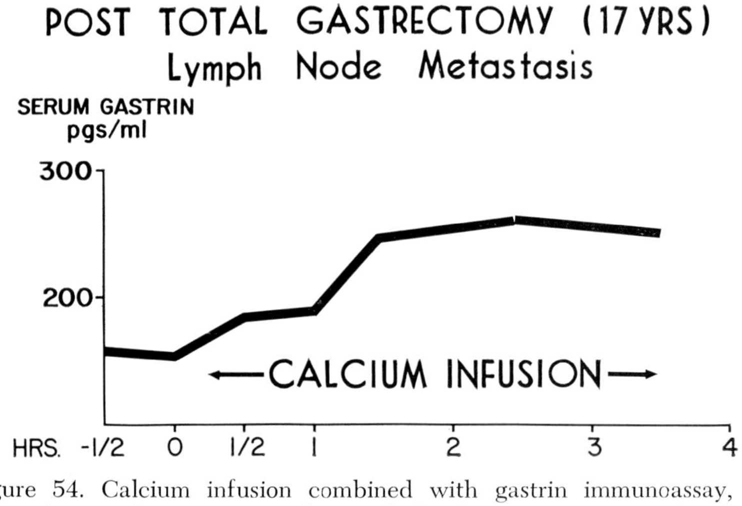

Figure 54. Calcium infusion combined with gastrin immunoassay, 17-½ years after total gastrectomy showed little change, suggesting the absence of active gastrin-producing tumors.

same holds true for the cell responsible for the diarrheogenic syndrome. Embryologically it is not entirely out of reason to assume that the pluripotential cell which is involved in the development of the duodenum, gastric antrum, gallbladder, and ducts as well as the dorsal bud of the pancreas can produce an excess of hormone when involved as an islet cell tumor. Gastrin and secretin should be the two other most likely hormones other than insulin, since they arise from either the antrum or the duodenum. However, other hormones such as serotonin, MSH, and ACTH have also been associated with the non-beta islet cell tumor.

Grossly, the non-beta islet cell tumors have tended to be relatively larger than the beta cell tumors. This is particularly true for the tumors associated with the diarrheogenic syndrome. They are located throughout the gland, so that blind resection of the body and tail gives only a two thirds chance of removing the source of the potent gastric secretagogue arising from the pancreas. They also commonly occur as diffuse microadenomatosis which cannot be positively identified at the time of surgery. About 7 per cent occur within the wall of the duodenum either as discrete nodules or by microscopic examination of a cross section of the duodenal wall. Metastasis to the adjacent lymph nodules or liver occurs in approximately two out of three cases. This high incidence of malignancy with the multisource for the production of excess gastrin production makes removal of all the gastric secreting surface the most logical initial surgical procedure if the patient is to be insured of a long-term relief of symptoms. It would appear, however, that when the non-beta islet cell tumor occurs within the wall of the duodenum there is a greater chance that this may be only lesion present unless local metastasis has already occurred.

Bloodworth and Elliott,[189] in a study of pancreatic islet cell lesions, emphasized how frequently they showed a similar morphologic picture whether benign or malignant. It is usually necessary to find direct extension beyond the capsule of the pancreas or metastasis to prove the malignant potential of the tumor. Microscopically the islet cell tumors tend to be of two patterns. One is called the "ribbon" or trabecular pattern. The other common type is a medullary tumor which sometimes shows a "tubule" or "rosette" formation. The histologic pattern is not correlated with either malignancy or the functional capacity of the tumor. It is very doubtful if a difference can be noticed between those tumors providing gastrin and those associated with hyperparalleyroidism and diarrhea (Fig. 55).

On occasion the ulcerogenic syndrome has existed without proof of an islet cell tumor; however, there was evidence of extensive hyperplasia and neoformation of islets from proliferating tubules. Brown and Still[497] reported a case of the ulcerogenic syndrome associated with nesidioblastosis of the islets with proliferation of the islets and intercalated duct cells. They suggested that an extrapancreatic agent may be responsible for such histological changes in the pancreas leading to an excessive production of gastrin and an ulcerogenic syndrome.

The islet cell tumors associated with watery diarrhea, hypokalemia, and achlorhydria tend to be larger than the ulcerogenic islet cell tumor. However, the incidence of malignancy in the less

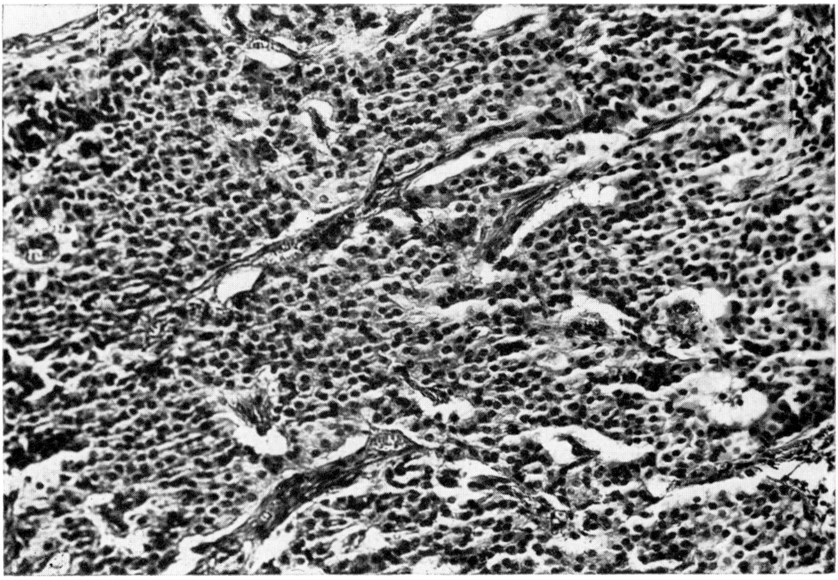

Figure 55. A typical islet cell tumor pattern. They commonly have ribbon or alveolar patterns and frequently represent carcinoid tumor.

than 50 cases reported similar to that of the ulcerogenic tumor. The microscopic studies have failed to yield the identification of the cell in these tumors responsible for the syndrome. Immunologic technics, electronmicroscopy, and increased interest in the potential of islet cell tumors to produce a variety of important clinical syndromes will eventually clarify the cell of origin of the various syndromes which have defied identification for so long.

The beta and alpha cell apparently have been ruled out but the delta cell or an "X" cell remains to be incriminated in the ulcerogenic as well as the diarrheogenic islet cell tumor syndrome.

REFERENCES

1955

1. Zollinger, R. M., and Ellison, E.: Primary peptic ulcerations of the jejunum associated with islet cell tumors of the pancreas. *Ann Surg, 142:*709, 1955.

1956

2. Eiseman, B., and Maynard, R. M.: A non-insulin producing islet cell adenoma associated with progressive peptic ulceration. *Gastroenterology, 31:*296, 1956
3. Ellison, E.: The ulcerogenic tumor of the pancreas. *Surgery, 40:*147, 1956.

1957

4. Busteed, F., and Speir, E.: A case of islet cell carcinoma of the pancreas, associated with peptic ulceration of the jejunum. *Arch Surg, 74:*703, 1957.
5. Castleman, B.: Case 43242. Case records of the Massachusetts General Hospital. *New Eng J Med, 256:*1153, 1957.
6. Donaldson, R. M., Jr.: Ulcerogenic tumor of the pancreas—a clinical note. *Bull Tufts-New Eng Med Cen, 3:*90, 1957.
7. Donaldson, R. M., Jr., Vom Eigen, P. R., and Dwight, R. W.: Gastric hypersecretion, peptic ulceration, and islet-cell tumor of the pancreas (the Zollinger-Ellison syndrome). *New Eng J Med, 257:*965, 1957.
8. Ellison, E. H., and Zollinger, R. M.: Ulcerogenic tumor of the pancreas. *Mod Med,* 87–90, 1957.
9. Fisher, E. R., and Flandreau, R. H.: Multiple endocrine tumors and peptic ulcer. *Gastroenterology, 32:*1075, 1957.
10. Ford, T., Jr., Jordan, G. L., Jr., Erickson, E., *et al.*: Recurrent gastrojejunal ulceration and islet cell carcinoma of the pancreas. *Arch Surg, 75:*272, 1957.

11. Priest, W. M., and Alexander, M. K.: Islet cell tumor of the pancreas with peptic ulceration, diarrhea and hypokalemia. *Lancet, 2:*1145, 1957.
12. Von Planta, V. F.: Nicht-insulinproduzierende Inselzellgeschwulst des pancreas und ulcus pepticum. Zollinger-Ellison syndrome. *Schweiz Med Wochensdr 87:*1272, 1957.
13. Zollinger, R. M.: The physiologic disturbances associated with pancreatic tumors. Proceedings 3rd National Cancer Conference, 779–80, 1957.

1958

14. Alvarez, W. C.: The Zollinger-Ellison syndrome; gastric hypersecretion, peptic ulceration, and an islet cell tumor of the pancreas. *Gastroenterology, 35:*109, 1958.
15. Cope, O., Keynes, W. M., Roth, S. I., *et al.:* Primary chief-cell hyperplasia of the parathyroid glands: a new entity in the surgery of hyperparathyroid:sm. *Ann Surg, 148:*375, 1958.
16. Gallert-Esquerdo, A.: Ulcerogenic tumor of pancreas. *Rev Esp Enferm Apar Dig, 17:*3, 1958.
17. Ghosh, M. N., and Schild, H. O.: Continuous recording of acid gastric secretion in the rat. *Brit J Pharmacol, 13:*54, 1958.
18. Hellstrom, J.: Hyperparathyroidism and gastroduodenal ulcer. *Acta Chir Scand, 116:*207, 1958–59.
19. Leger, L., and Cazes, B.: Hypersecretion gastrique, ulcere digestif, tumeur Langerhansienne non insulinogene syndrome de Zollinger et Ellison. *Presse Med, 66:*958, 1958.
20. MacKenzie, W. C., Norvell, S. T., Jr., Mathews, B. L., *et al.:* Islet cell tumours and peptic ulcers; a report of two cases of the Zollingèr-Ellison syndrome. *Canad J Surg, 2:*6, 1958.
21. Maynard, E. P., III, and Point, W. W.: Steatorrhea associated with ulcerogenic tumor of the pancreas. *Am J Med, 25:*456, 1958.
22. Oberhelman, H. A., Jr., Nelsen, T. S., and Dragstedt, L. R.: Peptic ulcer associated with tumors of the pancreas. *Arch Surg, 77:*402, 1958.
23. Schlumberger, M. D.: Ulcerogenic cerebral lesions and pancreatic tumors. *J Arkansas Med Soc, 54:*305, 1958.
24. Thistlewaite, J. R., and Horwitz, A.: Ulcerogenic islet cell tumors of the pancreas. *Postgrad Med, 24:*599, 1958.
25. Verner, J., and Morrison, A.: Islet cell tumor and a syndrome of refractory watery diarrhea and hypokalemia. *Am J Med, 25:*374, 1958.
26. Zollinger, R. M.: Evaluation of the surgical treatment of intractable duodenal ulcer. *Arch Int Med, 102:*607, 1958.
27. Zollinger, R. M., and Elliott, D. W.: Pancreatic endocrine function and peptic ulceration. *Gastroenterology, 37:*419, 1958.

28. Zollinger, R. M., and McPherson, R. C.: Ulcerogenic tumors of the pancreas. *Am J Surg, 95:*359, 1958.
29. Zubrod, C. G.: Acromegaly, jejunal ulcers and hypersecretion of gastric juice: clinico-pathological conference at the National Institutes of Health. *Ann Int Med, 49:*1389, 1958.

1959

30. Billington, B. P.: Gastric secretion and the Zollinger-Ellison syndrome. *Lancet, 1:*886, 1959.
31. Cernik, V. P.: The existence and etiology of the Zollinger-Ellison syndrome. *Plzen Lek Sbor, 8:*61, 1959.
32. Farrar, T., McBurney, R. P., and Sanders, R. L.: Recurrent stomal ulcer. Refractive to repeated operative procedures. An additional case of ulcerogenic tumor of the pancreas. *Am J Gastroent, 31:*64, 1959.
33. Friedell, H. V., and Rydell, J. R.: Ulcerogenic tumor of the pancreas. *Am J Gastroent, 31,* 58:1959.
34. Giec, L., Szpecht, J., and Zajusz, K.: (Zollinger-Ellison syndrome. Case report). *Pol Tyg Lek, 14:*1101, 1959.
35. Goulon, M., Mercier, J. N., Reilly, J., *et al.:* Langerhans carcinoma responsible for chronic diarrhea, severe hypokalemia with paralysis and hypoglycemia. Hypokalemia by transfer and by depletion. *Bull Mem Soc Med Hop,* 16, 1959.
36. Hendrick, J. M., David, J. S., and Shamblin, U. L., Jr.: Ulcerogenic tumors of the pancreas. *Am J Surg, 97:*92, 1959.
37. Hofbauer, K.: Zur diagnose des pankreasinselzelladenoms. (On the diagnosis of the pancreatic islet-cell adenoma). *Wien Med Wochenschr, 109:*708, 1959.
38. Knight, W.: Pancreatic component of peptic ulcer disease. *Amer J Dig Dis, 4:*910, 1959.
39. Pender, B.: Islet-cell tumour of the pancreas associated with peptic ulceration. *Lancet, 1:*123, 1959.
40. Peterva, V., and Cernik, L.: Kotazce existence a etiologie Zollingerova-Ellisonova syndromu. *Plzen Lek Sbor, 8:*61, 1959.
41. Summerskill, W. H. J.: The Zollinger-Ellison syndrome. *Mod Med,* 333, 1959.
42. Summerskill, W. H. J., and Oxon, D. M.: Malabsorption and jejunal ulceration due to gastric hypersecretion with pancreatic islet-cell hyperplasia. *Lancet,* 120, 1959.
43. Waddell, W. R., Leonsins, A. V., and Zuidema, G. D.: Gastric secretory and other laboratory studies on two patients with Zollinger-Ellison syndrome. *New Eng J Med, 260:*56, 1959.
44. Weber, J. M., Lewis, S., and Heasley, K. H.: Observations on the small bowel pattern associated with the Zollinger-Ellison syndrome. *Am J Roentgen, 72:*973, 1959.

45. Zollinger, R. M., and Elliott, D. W.: Pancreatic endocrine function and peptic ulceration. *Gastroenterology, 37:*419, 1959.

1960

46. Basian, H., and Zeifer, H. D.: Chronic recurrent peptic ulceration associated with multiple endocrinopathies. *Ann Surg, 152:*885, 1960.
47. Brusselmans, P.: Het syndroom van Zollinger-Ellison. *Belg Tyd Beneesk, 19:*281, 1960.
48. Carra, F.: I tumori ulcerogenici del pancreas. Sindrome di Zollinger ed Ellison. *Rec Prog Med (Peru), 28:*356, 1960.
49. Cawkell, W. I.: The Zollinger-Ellison syndrome. *New Zealand Med J, 59:*466, 1960.
50. Cazes, B.: [Ulcers associated with pancreatic tumors.] *Presse Med, 67:* 899, 1960.
51. Chvojka, V. E.: Islet-cell tumors and peptic ulcers. Case report of Zollinger-Ellison syndrome. *Ann Int Med, 53:*1180, 1960.
52. Cooke, W. T., Fowler, D. I., Gaddie, R., *et al.:* Multiple endocrine adenoma syndrome. *Gut, 1:*71, 1960.
53. Craig, J. S., Anderson, J. R., and MacFarlane, P. S.: Islet cell tumors of the pancreas: With report of three cases. *Glasgow Med J, 31:* 296, 1960.
54. Demling, L.: Das Zollinger-Ellison syndrome. *Deutsch Med Wochenschr, 85:*889, 1960.
55. Desneux, J. J., Musin, L., Goffin, R., *et al.:* Notes sur un cas d'ulceres recidivants par syndrome de Zollinger-Ellison. *Acta Med Belg, 23:* 336, 1960.
56. Dubarry, J. J.: Ulceres duodenaux et pathologie pancreatique. *Rev Prat (Bordeaux), 11:*2527, 1960.
57. Editorial: An expanding syndrome. *Lancet, 2:*137, 1960.
58. Elliott, D. W., and Zollinger, R. M.: Complications of pancreatic surgery. In Artz, C. P. and Hardy, J. D. (Eds.): Complications in surgery and their management. Philadelphia: Saunders, 699–733, 1960.
59. Fisher, E. R., and Hicks, J.: Further pathologic observations on the syndrome of peptic ulcer and multiple endocrine tumor. *Gastroenterology, 38:*458, 1960.
60. Frame, B. and Haubrich, W. S.: Peptic ulcer and hyperparathyroidism. A survey of 300 ulcer patients. *Arch Int Med, 105:*436, 1960.
61. Franksson, C., Hellstrom, J., Hultquist, G., *et al.:* Primary chief-cell hyperplasia of the parathyroids, and islet cell hyperplasia and adenomata of the pancreas associated with gastro-duodenal-jejunal ulcer. *Acta Chir Scand, 118:*270, 1960.
62. Gerber, B. C., Aberdeen, S. D., and Shields, T. W.: Simultaneous

duodenal carcinoid and non-beta cell tumors of the pancreas. Two tumors of high ulcerogenic potential. *Arch Surg, 81:*379, 1960.

63. Gibson, J. B., and Welbourn, R. B.: Islet cell tumors and peptic ulceration. *Postgrad Med J, 36:*154, 1960.
64. Gondard, M. L.: Tumeurs insulaires du pancreas non insulinogenes et syndrome de Zollinger-Ellison. *Arch Mal Appar Dig, 49:*1217, 1960.
65. Goulon, M., Mercier, J. N., Reilly, J., *et al.:* Carcinome Langerhansien responsable d'hypersecretion gastrique acide, de diarrhee chronique, d'hypokaliemie severe avec paralysies et d'hypoglycemie. *Sem Hop, 36:*172, 1960.
66. Gray, S. J.: The adrenal glands and peptic ulcer. *Gastroenterology, 39:*553, 1960.
67. Gregory, R. A., Tracy, H. J., French, J. M., *et al.:* Extraction of a gastrin-like substance from a pancreatic tumor in a case of Zollinger-Ellison syndrome. *Lancet, 1:*1045, 1960.
68. Leffkowitz, M., Laundau, B., and Boss, J. H.: Insulinoma associated with peptic ulcers. Report of a case. *Gastroent (Basal), 93:*157, 1960.
69. Leger, L., Premont, M., and Guyet-Roussett, Mme.: Les carcinomes Langerhansiens. *J Chir (Paris), 80:*291, 1960.
70. Lehoczky, D., Balazs, M., Kardos, E., *et al.:* Pankreas szigetadenoma es peptikus fekely cgyuttes clofordulsas: Zollinger-Ellison syndroma. *Orv Het, 102:*2520, 1960.
71. Loughridge, J. S., Neill, D. W., and Willis, J.: Zollinger-Ellison syndrome. Report of a case. *Brit J Surg, 48:*158, 1960.
72. MacKenzie, W. C., and Norvell, S. T., Jr.: Islet cell tumours and peptic ulcers. *J Roy Coll Surg (Edinburgh) 5:*191, 1960.
73. Marner, I. L., Mathiesen, F. R., and Tobiassen, G.: Gastro-intestinal acidity in the Strom-Zollinger-Ellison syndrome. *Acta Chir Scand, 119:*422, 1960.
74. Murphy, R. T., Goodsitt, E., Morales, H., *et al.:* Peptic ulceration with associated endocrine tumors. Collective review and report of a case. *Am J Surg, 100:*764, 1960.
75. Osborne, M. P., Brown, M. E., and LeCompte, P. M.: Ulcerogenic non-beta cell pancreatic islet carcinoma. Studies on the extraction and assay of a possible gastric secretagogue. *Am J Surg, 100:*48, 1960.
76. Pernod, R., Bader, J. P., Martin, J. C., *et al.:* Le syndrome de Zollinger et Ellison. A propos d'un cas opere et suivi depuis huit mois. *Mem Acad Chir, 86:*364, 1960.
77. Rawson, A. B., England, M. T., Gillam, G. G., *et al.:* Zollinger-Ellison syndrome with diarrhea and malabsorption. Observations on a patient before and after pancreatic islet cell tumor removal without resort to gastric surgery. *Lancet, 2:*131, 1960.

78. Reyl-Stelle, J. D. R., and Fernandez, G. A.: Un caso de ulceras multiples duodeno. *Rev Esp Enferm Apar Dig, 19:*1011, 1960.
79. Roth, J. L. A., and Vilardell, F.: Pituitary adenoma and peptic ulcer disease. A review of the literature. *Gastroenterology, 39:*558, 1960.
80. Rudolf, L. E., Dammin, G. F., and Moore, F. D.: Intractable peptic ulcer and endocrine adenomas with pituitary amphophilic hyperplasia. *Surgery, 48:*170, 1960.
81. Sanchez, G. C., and Sommers, S. C.: Peptic ulcer diathesis with a mixed adenocarcinoma of the pancreas. Case report. *Gastroenterology, 38:*467, 1960.
82. Schindler, R., and DeOliveira, C. A.: Sindrome de "sprue nao tropical" e hiperplasia gastrica e duodenal, com ulceracoes do jejuno, num caso de carcinoma das ilhotas de Langerhans (Sindrome de ma absorcao, associada a sindrome de Zollinger-Ellison). *Gastroent (Brasil), 12:*17, 1960.
83. Schlaeger, R., LeMay, M., and Wermer, P.: Upper gastrointestinal tract alterations in adenomatosis of the endocrine glands. *Radiology, 75:*517, 1960.
84. Scott, H. W., Jr., Herrington, J. L., Jr., Edwards, L. W., *et al.:* Results of vagotomy and antral resection in surgical treatment of duodenal ulcer. *Gastroenterology, 39:*590, 1960.
85. Sieracki, J., Marshall, R. B., and Horn, R. C., Jr.: Tumors of the pancreatic islets. *Cancer, 13:*349, 1960.
86. Slama, R.: Le syndrome de Zollinger-Ellison. *La Vie Med, 41:*306, 1960.
87. Spiro, H. M.: Hyperparathyroidism, parathyroid "adenomas," and peptic ulcer. *Gastroenterology, 39:*544, 1960.
88. Symposium: Discussion of symposium on adenomas of endocrine glands and peptic ulcer. *Gastroenterology, 39:*566, 1960.
89. Vilardell, F.: Ulcera peptic y adenomas multiples endocrinos. *Rev Clin Esp, 77:*382, 1960.
90. Wilkinson, L. H., Simms, A. G., II, Floyd, V. T., *et al.:* Multiple duodenal ulcers with fatal hemorrhage. *Arch Surg, 80:*753, 1960.
91. Zollinger, R. M.: Endocrine adenomas and peptic ulcer. With special reference to pancreatic adenomas. *Gastroenterology, 39:*541, 1960.
92. Zollinger, R. M.: Symposium: Adenomas of endocrine glands and peptic ulcer. With special reference to pancreatic adenomas. *Gastroenterology, 39:*541, 1960.
93. Zollinger, R. M.: Surgical clinicopathological conference. Mass Gen Hosp. *New Eng J Med, 263:*1132, 1960.
94. Zollinger, R. M., and Craig, T. V.: Endocrine tumors and peptic ulcer. *Am J Med, 29:*761, 1960.
95. Zollinger, R. M., and Craig, T. V.: Ulcerogenic tumors of the pancreas. *Am J Surg, 99:*424, 1960.

1961

96. Arean, V.: Tumores endocrinos del pancreas. *Rev Clin Esp, 83:*185, 1961.
97. Aron, E., Leger, L., and Fekete, F.: Ulcere digestif et tumeur Langerhansienne (Syndrome de Zollinger et Ellison). *Presse Med, 69:* 143, 1961.
98. Baker, R. L.: Familial adenomatosis of endocrine glands. Presentation of a new family. *Northwest Med, 60:*905, 1961.
99. Batko, B., and Nekrat, J.: Przpadek zespotu Zollingera-Ellisona. *Pol Tyg Led, 16:*1157, 1961.
100. Borg, I., Soderstrom, J., and Haeger, K.: Pancreatic islet tumors and peptic ulcer. *Acta Chir Scand, 120:*422, 1961.
101. Case 48: Ulcerogenic tumor of the pancreas. In Glenn, F. and Wantz, G. E., Jr.: Problems in surgery from surgical grand rounds at The New York Hospital-Cornell Medical Center. St. Louis: Mosby, 181, 1961.
102. Castleman, B. (Ed.): Case records of the Massachusetts General Hospital (Case 62–1961). *New Eng J Med, 265:*439, 1961.
103. Cattan, R., Frumusan, P., Hivet, M., *et al.:* Syndrome de Zollinger-Ellison. Deux nouveaux cas. *Bull Soc Med Hop (Paris), 77:*914, 1961.
104. Dorken, von H.: (Some data on 280 patients with pancreatic tumors). *Gastroent (Germany), 102:*47, 1961.
105. Elliott, D. W., Taft, D. A., Passaro, E. J., Jr., *et al.:* Pancreatic influence on gastric secretions. *Surgery, 50:*126, 1961.
106. Fahrlander, V. H., Nissen, R., Scheidegger, S., *et al.:* Nicht-insulinproduzierendes pancreasadenom mit ulcus duodeni (Zollinger-Ellison syndrome). *Schweiz Med Wochenschr, 91:*1288, 1961.
107. Fegiz, G.: La sindrome di Zollinger-Ellison. *Prog Med (Naples), 17:* 211, 1961.
108. French, J. M., and Sircus, W.: The Zollinger-Ellison syndrome. In Card, W. I.: *Gastroenterology.* 178–198, 1961.
109. Gandhi, M. J.: Ulcerogenic tumors of pancreas (Zollinger-Ellison syndrome). *Indian J Med Sci, 15:*476, 1961.
110. Grossman, M. I., Tracy, H. J., and Gregory, R. A.: II Islolation of a gastrin-like substance from the primary and secondary tumors. *Gastroenterology, 41:*87, 1961.
111. Hivet, M., Julien, C., and Levame, Mme.: Cinq observations due syndrome de Zollinger-Ellison. *Rev Med Chir (Paris), 36:*257, 1961.
112. Joyeux, R., Colin, R., and Gondard, L.: Ulcere peptique recidivant avec tumeur insulaire non insulinogene (Syndrome de Zollinger-Ellison). *Montpellier Med, 59:*135, 1961.
113. Julien, C.: Le syndrome de Zollinger et Ellison. *Rev Med Chir (Paris), 36:*266, 1961.

114. Marcussen, J. M.: Strom-Zollinger-Ellison syndrome. *Nord Med, 66:* 1017, 1961.
115. Markowitz, A. M., Slanetz, C. A., Jr., and Frantz, V. K.: Functioning islet cell tumors of the pancreas. *Ann Surg, 154:*877, 1961.
116. Marks, I. N., Selzer, G., Louw, J. H., *et al.:* Zollinger-Ellison syndrome in a Bantu woman with isolation of gastrin-like substance from the primary and secondary tumors. *Gastroenterology, 41:*77, 1961.
117. Martin, E., Potet, F., Bader, J-P., *et al.:* Trois cas de cancer pancreatique endocrine non insulinogene. Rapports avec le syndrome de Zollinger-Ellison. Constations histologiques particulieres. *Arch Anat Path, 9:*203, 1961.
118. Mogena, H. G., and Alvarez, F. A.: La ulcera gastroduodenal de origen endocrino. *Rev Clin Esp, 8:*387, 1961.
119. Monaco, A. P., Lythgoe, J. P., and Waddell, W. R.: Immunological study in the Zollinger-Ellison syndrome. *Lancet, 2:*1016, 1961.
120. Oberhelman, H. A., Jr., Nelsen, T. S., Johnson, A. N., Jr., *et al.:* Ulcerogenic tumors of the duodenum. *Ann Surg, 153:*241, 1961.
121. Poth, E. J., Cleveland, B. R., and Nash, J. B.: Pancreatic secretion and peptic ulcer formation. *Amer J Surg, 101:*154, 1961.
122. Potter, J. F., and Sabesin, S. M.: Intractable peptic ulceration associated with islet cell carcinoma of the pancreas (Zollinger-Ellison syndrome) and with endocrine adenomatosis. *Ann Surg, 154:*885, 1961.
123. Roselli, A., and Paulino, F.: Sindrome de Zollinger-Ellison. (Relato de um caso). *Hospital (Rio), 60:*209, 1961.
124. Roux, M., and Jureau, J.: Ulcere due "genu superius" et pa creas aberrant de la paroi du deuxieme duodenum. *Presse Med, 69:* 2141, 1961.
125. Saint, E. G., Finlay-Jones, R., and Stewart, H. H.: Familial endocrine adenomatosis with ulcerogenic tumor of the pancreas. *Aust Ann Med, 10:*308, 1961.
126. Schmid, J. R., Labhart, A., and Rossier, P. H.: Relationship of multiple endocrine adenomas to the syndrome of ulcerogenic islet cell adenomas (Zollinger-Ellison). Occurrence of both syndromes in one family. *Am J Med, 31:*343, 1961.
127. Silen, W.: Ulzerogene tumoren des pankreas (Zollinger-Ellison syndrome). *Schweiz Rund Med, 50:*1207, 1961.
128. Smith, R.: Pancreatic neoplasms. *Proc Roy Soc Med, 54:*1124, 1961.
129. Summerskill, W. H. J., Code, C. F., Hallenbeck, G. A., *et al.:* Intractable peptic ulcer in hereditary endocrine-ulcer disease. Gastrin content of endocrine tissues. *Proc Mayo Clin, 36:*611, 1961.
130. Terrasse, J., Lauras, H., Moinade, S., *et al.:* Un diagnostic errone de syndrome de Zollinger-Ellison. *Rev Prac, 11:*2541, 1961.
131. Wilder, W. T., Frame, B., and Haubrich, W. S.: Peptic ulcer in pri-

mary hyperparathyroidism. An analysis of 52 cases. *Ann Int Med, 55:*885, 1961.

1962

132. Anton, A. T.: Non-beta islet cell carcinoma of the pancreas. *Ohio Med J, 58:*1376, 1962.
133. Auguste, C., Ribet, M., Gerard, A., *et al.:* Developpement d'un cancer du pancreas un an apres exerese d'un adenome brunnerien de l'antre. *Arch Mal Appar Dig, 51:*1594, 1962.
134. Berdjis, C. C.: Pluriglandular syndrome. Multiple endocrine adenomas in man. *Oncologia (Basel), 15:*288, 1962.
135. Block, M. A., Smith, R. F., Haubrich, W. S., *et al.:* Surgical problems in management of islet-cell tumors with gastric hypersecretion. *Arch Surg, 85:*270, 1962.
136. Campbell, A. C. P., Gowenlock, A. H., Plat, D. S., *et al.:* A 5-hydroxy-tryptophan-secreting carcinoid tumor. *Gut, 3:*61, 1962.
137. Catchpole, R. B.: The role of the pancreas in gastric secretion. *Gut, 3:*336, 1962.
138. Code, C. F., Hallenbeck, G. A., and Summerskill, W. H. J.: Extraction of a gastric secretagogue from primary and metastatic islet cell tumors in three cases of Zollinger-Ellison syndrome. *J Surg Res, 2:*136, 1962.
139. Costescu, N.: Association of ulcerous disease with pancreatic tumor of the non-insulinogenic type (Zollinger-Ellison syndrome). *Med Int (Rumania), 14:*81, 1962.
140. Danowski, T. S., Mateer, F. M., and Longabaugh, E. E.: Endocrine adenomatosis. *Acta Med Scand, 172:*559, 1962.
141. Darvish, N., Keister, S. R., and Brockmyer, M. L.: Zollinger-Ellison syndrome with pneumopericardium and cholecystoduodenal fistula. *Penn Med J, 65:*703, 1962.
142. Davis, C. E., Jr., Smith, P., Jr., and Davalos, X. S.: Ulcerogenic tumor of the pancreas. *Ann Surg, 155:*669, 1962.
143. Dubarry, J. J.: Ulceres multiples duodeno-jejunaux a perforations interatives. Syndrome de Zollinger-Ellison probable. *Presse Med, 70:*24, 1962.
144. Dubarry, J. J., and Bernard, J-P.: Recent acquisitions in gastro-enterology. *J Med Bordeaux, 193:*1225, 1962.
145. Edmeads, J. G., Mathews, R. E., McPhedran, N. T., *et al:* Diarrhea caused by pancreatic islet cell tumors. *Canad Med Ass J, 86:*847, 1962.
146. Feyrter, F.: Uber den derzeitigen stand der lehre von den peripheren endokrinen (parakrinen) drusen. *Acta Neurol (Austria), 25:*63, 1962.
147. Friesen, S. R., Tracy, H. J., and Gregory, R. A.: Mechanism of the gastric hypersecretion in the Zollinger-Ellison syndrome. Successful

extraction of gastrin-like activity from metastases and primary pancreatico-duodenal islet cell carcinoma. *Ann Surg, 155:*167, 1962.

148. Fried, L.: Der ulzerogene pankreastumor-Das Zollinger-Ellison-syndrom. *Radiol Diag (Hungary), 3:*463, 1962.
149. Gendreau, C.: Le syndrome de Zollinger-Ellison. *Union Med (Canada), 91:*1507, 1962.
150. Gesztesi, T., and Wallacher, L.: Ulcerogenic tumor of the pancreas. Zollinger-Ellison syndrome. *Orv Hetil, 103:*1132, 1962.
151. Greider, M. H., Zollinger, R. M., Elliott, D. W., *et al.:* Electron microscopic study of ulcerogenic tumors of the pancreas. Fifth International Congress for Electron Microscopy. New York: Academic Press, 1962.
152. Gutch, C. F., and Kisner, P.: Islet cell tumor, diarrhea and hypopotasemia. (The Zollinger-Ellison syndrome) *Nebraska Med J, 47:* 119, 1962.
153. Hansen, J. R.: Islet cell carcinoma of the pancreas. *Ann Surg, 155:* 518, 1962.
154. Haubrich, W. S., O'Neill, F. S., and Block, M. A.: Observations on steatorrhea associated with gastric hypersecretion and pancreatic islet cell neoplasm. *Ann Int Med, 56:*302, 1962.
155. Hershfield, B. M., and Janis, R.: Myocardial infarction with multiple endocrine adenomatosis and two primary carcinomas. *Jewish Mem Hosp Bull (NY), 6–7:*167, 1962.
156. Joyeux, R., and Colin, R.: Le probleme therapeutique des ulceres peptiques recidivants. A propos du syndrome Zollinger-Ellison. *J Chir (Paris), 83:*547, 1962.
157. Julien, C., Bader, J-P., Lambling, A., *et al.:* Etude clinique du syndrome de Zollinger-Ellison. A propos de quatre observations personnelles. *Arch Mal App Dig, 51:*249, 1962.
158. Lambling, A.: L'hypergastrie acido-peptique pancreatogene du syndrome de Zollinger-Ellison et de ses relations avec la maladie ulcereuse. *Arch Mal App Dig, 51:*331, 1962.
159. Lambling, A., Bader, J-P., Bernier, J. J., *et al.:* L'hypersecretion chlorhydropeptique de l'estomac dans le syndrome de Zollinger-Ellison. *Arch Mal App Dig, 51:*263, 1962.
160. Lauste, L. W.: Zollinger-Ellison syndrome. *Proc Roy Soc Med, 55:* 806, 1962.
161. Lawrie, R. S., Williamson, A. W. R., and Hunt, J. N.: Zollinger-Ellison syndrome treated with Polidine methyl methosulphate. *Lancet, 1:* 1002, 1962.
162. Lucerga, B. B., and Lazaro, A. R. D.: Ulcera peptica asociada con tumores endocrinos multiples. *Rev Clin Esp, 84:*73, 1962.

163. MacKenzie, W. C.: Islet cell lesions of the pancreas. *West Indian Med J, 2:*161, 1962.
164. Maks, S. W., and Saul, R. H.: Zollinger-Ellison syndrome. Report of a case. *Portland Clin Bull, 14:*65, 1962.
165. Martin, E. T., and Potet, F.: Anatomie pathologique du syndrome de Zollinger-Ellison. *Arch. Mal App Dig, 51:*281, 1962.
166. Mathews, R. E., Bett, H. D., Edmeads, J. G., *et al.:* Physiological effects of extracts of a diarrhea-producing nonbeta islet cell tumor of the pancreas. *Surg Gynec Obst, 115:*490, 1962.
167. Meeroff, M., and Feldfeber, B.: Ulcera peptica asociada a adenomas glandulares. Syndrome de Zollinger-Ellison. *Prensa Med Argent, 49:*831, 1962.
168. Mieher, W. C., Jr., Hartsock, R. J., Goekas, M. C., *et al.:* Peptic ulcer as a manifestation of familial polyendocrine disease. *JAMA, 179:* 854, 1962.
169. Moldawer, M.: Multiple endocrine tumors and Zollinger-Ellison syndrome in families. One or two syndromes? A report of two new families. *Metabolism, 11:*153, 1962.
170. Morrison, A. B., Rawson, A. J., and Fitts, W. T., Jr.: The syndrome of refractory watery diarrhea and hypokalemia in patients with a noninsulin-secreting islet cell tumor. A further case study and review of the literature. *Am J Med, 32:*119, 1962.
171. Orfali, J., and Martin, E.: Un nouveau cas de tumeur pancreatique ulcerogene. Syndrome de Zollinger-Ellison. *Acad Chir, 88:*334, 1962.
172. Pearl, M. A., Sternberg, W. H., and Dingman, J. F.: Unusual cases of hyperparathyroidism. *Arch Int Med, 110:*481, 1962.
173. Pernod, M. J., Mercadier, M., and Hepp, J.: A propos du traitement chirurgical du syndrome de Zollinger-Ellison. *Arch Mal App Dig, 51:*323, 1962.
174. Santangelo, U.: La sindrome di Zollinger-Ellison. *Rif Med, 76:*667, 1962.
175. Schmitz, E. J.: The Zollinger-Ellison syndrome. In Harkins, H. and Nyhus, L. (Eds.): *Surgery of the Stomach and Duodenum,* 1962.
176. Shay, H., Chey, W. Y., Koide, S. M., *et al.:* Mechanism of the disordered physiology involved in the Zollinger-Ellison syndrome. Report of a case. *Am J Dig Dis, 7:*401, 1962.
177. Singleton, A. O., Jr., and Cunningham, P.: Islet cell tumors of the pancreas. *Ann Surg, 155:*663, 1962.
178. Smith, R.: Debatable issues in biology and pancreatic surgery. The Zollinger-Ellison syndrome. *Mod Trends Surg, 1:*58, 1962.
179. Stevenson, C., Acchiardo, S., Barzelatto, J., *et al.:* Sindrome de Zollinger-Ellison. *Rev Med Chile, 90:*273, 1962.
180. Thiery, J-P., and Bader, J-P.: Etude cytologique d'une tumeur de

pancreas (Syndrome de Zollinger-Ellison). Observation en contraste de phase et en microscopic electronique. *Arch Mal App Dig, 51:*301, 1962.

181. Williams, E. D., and Celestin, L. R.: The association of bronchial carcinoid and pluriglandular adenomatosis. *Thorax, 17:*120, 1962.
182. Wilson, S. D., Hurley, J. D., and Ellison, E. H.: Heterologous transplantation and growth in tissue culture of ulcerogenic tumor cells from patients with the Zollinger-Ellison syndrome. *Lancet, 2:* 1307, 1962.
183. Zollinger, R. M., and Elliott, D. W.: Ulcerogenic tumors of the pancreas and management of pancreatitis. *Med Sci, 12:*857, 1962.
184. Zollinger, R. M., Elliott, D. W., Endahl, G. L., *et al.:* Origin of the ulcerogenic hormone in endocrine-induced ulcer. *Ann Surg, 156:* 570, 1962.

1963

185. Angervall, L., Dotevall, G., Lehmann, K-E., *et al.:* Zollinger-Ellison syndrome: Report of a case. *Gastroenterology, 44:*512, 1963.
186. Bader, J-P., Laudat, P., Dubrasquet, M., *et al.:* Pouvoir secretagogue (PSU) d'une fraction d'urines humaines vis-a-vis de l'estomac du rat. *Rend Soc Biol (Paris), 157:*1390, 1963.
187. Barre, C.: Endocrinopathies et ulceres duodenaux. *Prog Med (France), 91:*64, 1963.
188. Bernstein, E. F., McFee, A. S., Goodale, R. L., Jr., *et al.:* Treatment of postgastrectomy stomal ulcer by gastric freezing. *Arch Surg, 87:* 13, 1963.
189. Bloodworth, J. M. B., Jr., and Elliott, D. W.: The histochemistry of pancreatic islet cell lesions. *JAMA, 183:*1011, 1963.
190. Bonfils, S., Bader, J-P., Dubrasquet, M., *et al.:* Despitage, dans les urines humaines, de substances excitant la secretion gastrique du rat. *Comp Rend Soc Biol (Paris), 157:*259, 1963.
191. Brusselmans, P.: Het syndroom van Zollinger-Ellison. *Belg Tyd Geneesk (Louvaine), 19:*281, 1963.
192. Bullock, R. G.: Report of a case of the Zollinger-Ellison syndrome associated with multiple endocrine adenomas. *Med Ann DC, 32:* 185, 1963.
193. Campuzano, M.: Functional islet cell tumors of the pancreas. II. Case of ulcerogenic tumor with hyperinsulinism. *Rev Invest Clin, 15:* 213, 1963.
194. Dejode, L. R., Howard, J. M., Yamulla, S., *et al.:* Recurrent peptic ulceration and gastric hypersecretion associated with islet cell hyperplasia of the pancreas. *Brit J Surg, 50:*790, 1963.
195. Deshpande, C. K., and Antani, D. U.: Zollinger-Ellison syndrome. *Indian J Path Bact, 6:*63, 1963.
196. Dotevalle, G., Lindell, S-E., and Westling, H.: Histamine studies in

a case of Zollinger-Ellison's syndrome. A preliminary report. *Acta Med Scand, 174:*325, 1963.

197. Elliott, D. W., Endahl, G. L., Knoernschild, H. E., *et al.:* Relation of antrum to pancreatic-induced gastric hypersecretion. *Surgery, 54:* 9, 1963.
198. Fiedler, Z., Lomsky, R., Groh., J., *et al.:* Surgical problems in endocrine-active tumors of the islands of Langerhans. *Sborn Ved Prac Lek Fak Karlov Univ, 6:*229, 1963.
199. Finlay, J. M., Mortimer, D. C., Vidinli, E. R., *et al.:* Coexistent Zollinger-Ellison syndrome (polyglandular endocrine adenomatosis) and renal tubular necrosis. A case report. *Gastroenterology, 44:*824, 1963.
200. Fox, N. M., Jr., Ferris, D. O., Moertel, C. G., *et al.:* Pseudocyst coexistent with pancreatic carcinoma. *Ann Surg, 158:*971, 1963.
201. Gendreau, C.: Zollinger-Ellison syndrome. Acquisitiones recentes. *Union Med (Canada), 92:*676, 1963.
202. Giordano, A.: Sindrome di Zollinger-Ellison. *Gaz Int Med Chir (Spain), 68:*1312, 1963.
203. Goodrick, W. I., and Dockerty, M. B.: Zollinger-Ellison syndrome. Associated gastric tumor showing islet-cell features. *Minnesota Med, 46:*634, 1963.
204. Greider, M. H., Elliott, D. W., and Zollinger, R. M.: An electron microscope study of islet cell adenomas. *JAMA, 186:*566, 1963.
205. Hallenbeck, G. A., Code, C. F., and Kennedy, J. C.: Effects of extracts of primary and metastatic pancreatic islet cell tumors on gastric secretion. *Gastroenterology, 44:*631, 1963.
206. Hardy, J. D.: Islet cell tumors. *Amer J Med Sci, 246:*124, 1963.
207. Hirschowitz, B. I., Schenker, S., and Boyette, J. D.: A highly active gastric secretagogue extracted from a metastasis of a Zollinger-Ellison syndrome tumor. Report of a case. *Am J Dig Dis, 8:*499, 1963.
208. Jackson, R. H., Blair, E. L., Dawson, P. J., *et al.:* Gastrin activity of tumor tissue in a child with the Zollinger-Ellison syndrome. *Lancet, 2:*908, 1963.
209. Jones, R.: The Zollinger-Ellison syndrome. Report of a case presenting with steatorrhea. *Aust New Zeal J Surg, 32:*274, 1963.
210. Jordan, G. L., Jr., Law, S. W., and Foster, R. P.: The management of patients with islet-cell carcinoma exhibiting the Zollinger-Ellison syndrome. *Am J Surg, 195:*80, 1963.
211. Judd, D. R., Heimburger, I. L., Vellios, F., *et al.:* Zollinger-Ellison syndrome in adolescents. *Surgery, 54:*673, 1963.
212. Katzka, I., and Glicken, J.: The Zollinger-Ellison syndrome. Report of a case with protein studies on the gastric juice. *Am J Dig Dis, 8:* 673, 1963.

213. Knudson, R. J., and Lynch, R. C.: Peptic ulceration associated with multiple endocrinologic abnormalities. Case report and review of literature. *Am Surg, 29:*117, 1963.
214. Leading Article: Zollinger-Ellison syndrome. *Lancet, 1:*367, 1963.
215. Leoni, E.: Ulcera gastro-duodenale e tumori insulari. Rapporti pathogenetici. *Gaz Int Med Chir (Spain), 68:*1096, 1963.
216. Mainetti, J. M., Iturriza, F. C., and Sori, N. R.: Sindrome de Zollinger-Ellison por hiperplasia difusa de celulas no beta. *El Dia Med, 35:* 80, 1963.
217. Martyn, J. W., and Welsh, W. K.: Non-insulin-producing islet cell tumors of the pancreas. A review of five cases including four with Zollinger-Ellison syndrome. *Canad J Surg, 6:*296, 1963.
218. Nemes, T., Salamon, A., and Rajkovits, K.: Pancreas tumorhoz tarsulo kulonos gyomerverses. *Magy Belorv Arch, 16:*156, 1963.
219. O'Flynn, W. R.: A case of the Zollinger-Ellison syndrome with associated splenomegaly. *Postgrad Med J, 39:*658, 1963.
220. Parker, P. E., Soergel, K., and Ellison, E. H.: Effects of excessive hydrochloric acid on canine gastrointestinal tract. *Surg Forum, 14:* 333, 1963.
221. Polacek, M. A., and Ellison, E. H.: A comparative study of parietal cell mass and distribution in normal stomachs, in stomachs with duodenal ulcer, and in stomachs of patients with pancreatic adenoma. *Surg Forum, 14:*313, 1963.
222. Rosenburg, S. A., and Buchman, J. J.: The problem of recurrent gastrojejunal ulcer. *Am J Surg, 195:*680, 1963.
223. Schindler, R.: On hypertrophic glandular gastritis, hypertrophic gastropathy and parietal cell mass. *Gastroenterology, 45:*77, 1963.
224. Shieber, W.: Insulin-producing Zollinger-Ellison tumor. *Surgery, 54:* 448, 1963.
225. Sohn, E., Ryoo, U., Choi, H., *et al.:* Zollinger-Ellison syndrome. A case report and review of the literature. *J Korean Med Ass, 6:* 1279, 1963.
226. Soliani, F.: La sindrome di Zollinger-Ellison. *Policlin Sez Prat (Rome), 70:*719, 1963.
227. Spencer, S. S., and Summerskill, W. H. J.: Malabsorption induced by gastric hypersecretion due to ectopic islet cell adenoma. *Am J Gastroent, 39:*26, 1963.
228. Vichtomova, T. K.: [A rare case of adenomas of the four endocrine glands]. *Probl Endokr Gormonoter, 9:*105, 1963.
229. Wermer, P.: Endocrine adenomatosis and peptic ulcer in a large kindred. Inherited multiple tumors and mosaic pleiotropism in man. *Am J Med, 35:*205, 1963.
230. Wiederanders, R. E., and Classen, K. L.: Endocrine associated peptic ulcer. *Am J Surg, 106:*70, 1963.

231. Wilbur, B. C., Lee, R. H., and Jamplis, R. W.: Ulcerogenic tumors of the pancreas. Report of two cases and suggested treatment. *Surg Clin N Am, 43:*1343, 1963.

232. Wruble, L. D., Bennett, L. D., Davis, J., *et al.:* Zollinger-Ellison syndrome. Surgical removal of parietal cell mass with preservation of antrum and pylorus, ileocolonic transplant and resultant achlorhydria. *Ann Surg, 158:*270, 1963.

233. Zollinger, R. M.: Observations on the relationship of the pancreas to peptic ulcer. *Bull New York Acad Med, 39:*617, 1963.

234. Zollinger, R. M.: Special comment: The Zollinger-Ellison syndrome. In Harkins, H., and Nyhus, L. (Eds.): *Surgery of the Stomach and Duodenum.* Boston: Little, Brown, 252–53, 1963.

235. Zollinger, R. M., Grant, G. N., Elliott, D. W., *et al.:* Ulcerogenic tumor of the pancreas. *Am Surg, 29:*751, 1963.

1964

236. Abowd, T. V., and Bartlett, R. H.: Peptic ulcer: Theory and therapy. *Univ Mich Med Cent J, 30:*91, 1964.

237. Amberg, J. R., Ellison, E. H., Wilson, S. D., *et al.:* Roentgenographic observations in the Zollinger-Ellison syndrome. *JAMA, 190:*185, 1964.

238. Bader, J-P., Potet, F. G., and Lambling, A.: Etude histologique des ilots de Langerhans non tumoraux dans le syndrome de Zollinger-Ellison. *Gastroenterologia (Basel), 102:*135, 1964.

239. Ballard, H. S., Frame, B., and Hartsock, R. J.: Familial multiple endocrine adenoma-peptic ulcer complex. *Medicine (Baltimore) 48:* 481, 1964.

240. Bank, S., and Marks, I. N.: Circulating gastric secretagogue in Zollinger-Ellison syndrome. *Lancet, 2:*1012, 1964. Letters to the Editor.

241. Bergan, T.: Pancreas-ventrikel-syndromet. Strom-Zollinger-Ellisons syndrom. *T Norske Leg, 84:*1468, 1964.

242. Bollack, C., Batzenschlager, A., Tuchmann, L., *et al.:* A propos d'un cas de syndrome de Zollinger-Ellison. *Lyon Chir, 60:* 500, 1964.

243. Brandstater, M., McCutcheon, A. D., Hamilton, N. T., *et al.:* The Zollinger-Ellison syndrome. *Med J Aust, 2:*177, 1964.

244. Bryant, L. R., Moore, T. C., Carney, E. K.: Islet cell adenomas of the duodenum with recurrent peptic ulceration (Zollinger-Ellison syndrome). *Ann Surg, 160:*104, 1964.

245. Burke, G., Finer, J. R., and Sandlow, L. J.: Ulcerogenic tumor of the pancreas and hyperparathyroidism. *Gastroenterology, 47:*88, 1964.

246. Caroli, J., and Julien, C.: Contribution to the study of diarrhea caused by hyperchlorhydria. Two personal observations of chronic diarrhea with gastric acid hypersecretion of the Zollinger-Ellison syndrome. *Rev Medicochir Mal Foie, 39:*265, 1964.

247. Christlieb, A. R., and Schuster, M. M.: Zollinger-Ellison syndrome. A clinical appraisal based on a review of the literature. *Arch Int Med, 114:*381, 1964.

248. Christlieb, A. R., Shende, M., and Schuster, M. M.: Zollinger-Ellison syndrome: Report of a case supporting the hypothesis of extra-pancreatic etiology. *Ann Int Med, 60:*1059, 1964.

249. Clarke, A. M., Glenn, A. I. M., and Illingworth, C.: Zollinger-Ellison syndrome treated without gastric surgery. *Lancet, 1:*1360, 1964.

250. Creamer, B.: Small-intestinal mucosal dynamics and the environment. *Brit Med J, 2:*1373, 1964.

251. Davidson, J. S.: Ulceration of the esophagus in association with a tumor of the pancreas. *J Thor Cardiovasc Surg, 48:*200, 1964.

252. DeBray, C., Bricaire, H., Hardouin, J-P., *et al.:* Adenoma parathyroidien avec lithiase renale associe a une adenomatose pancreatique non insulinogene hypersecretion gastrique et ulceres peptiques recidivants (Syndrome de Zollinger-Ellison). *Ann Endocrin (Paris), 25:*401, 1964.

253. Demling, L., Ottenjann, R., and Gebhardt, H.: Pankreas und peptisches Geschwur. *Gastroent (Basel), 102:*129, 1964.

254. DeMuth, W. E., Jr.: Zollinger-Ellison syndrome. *Arch Surg, 88:*244, 1964.

255. Ellison, E. H., and Wilson, S. D.: The Zollinger-Ellison syndrome. Reappraisal and evaluation of 260 registered cases. *Ann Surg, 160:* 512, 1964.

256. Enderlin, F.: Ulcerogene tumoren des pankreas praktisch-klinische aspekte. *Helv Chir Acta, 31:*294, 1964.

257. Erskine, J. M., Discussant. Oberhelman, H. A. and Nelsen, T. S.: Surgical consideration in the management of ulcerogenic tumors of the pancreas and duodenum. *Am J Surg, 108:*132, 1964.

258. Folch, M. G., Collmonegal, S., de Molina, C., *et al.:* Tumor ulcerogenico. Sindrome de Zollinger-Ellison producido por un tumor duodenal. *Med Clin Barcelona, 42:*277, 1964.

259. Garcia, E. L., Guedes, J. R., Berastequi, V. N., *et al.:* Commentarios sobre un caso de syndrome de Zollinger-Ellison. *Rev Clin Esp, 94:* 304, 1964.

260. Goodman, J. M.: Duodenal submucosal islet cell adenoma and chronic gastroduodenitis. *Am J Surg, 108:*726, 1964.

261. Gray, J.: Endocrinopathies and peptic ulcer. *Am J Dig Dis, 9:*279, 1964.

262. Gregory, R. A.: Gastrin and the Zollinger-Ellison syndrome. *Irish J Med Sci, 6:*443, 1964.

263. Gregory, R. A., and Tracy, H. J.: A note on the nature of the gastrin-like stimulant present in Zollinger-Ellison tumors. *Gut, 5:*115, 1964.

264. Greider, M. H., and Elliott, D. W.: Electron microscopy of human pancreatic tumors of islet cell origin. *Am J Path, 44:*663, 1964.
265. Hallenbeck, G. A.: Gastroenterology at the Surgical Forum in 1963: A review. *Gastroenterology, 46:*360, 1964.
266. Howe, C. T., Elliott, D. W., and Zollinger, R. M.: Histamine metabolism in pancreatic-induced hypersecretion. *Surg Forum, 15:* 368, 1964.
267. Huizenga, K. A., Goodrick, K. A., and Summerskill, W. H. J.: Peptic ulcer with islet cell tumor. A reappraisal. *Am J Med, 37:*564, 1964.
268. Ingram, P. W.: Multiple adenoma syndrome. *Proc Roy Soc Med, 57:* 1126, 1964.
269. James, A. H.: Gastric epithelium in the duodenum. *Gut, 5:*285, 1964.
270. Kolodny, H. D., and Griboff, S. I.: Multiple endocrine adenomatosis. *J Mt Sinai Hosp (NY), 31:*179, 1964.
271. Krivine, J-M, Hivet, M., and Levame, Mme.: Les tumeurs apparemment bénignes du duodénum. *Ann Chir, 18:*558, 1964.
272. LaBrie, H. J.: Ulcerogenic tumors of the pancreas (Zollinger-Ellison syndrome). *J Int Coll Surg, 42:*263, 1965.
273. Lai, K. S.: Studies on gastrin. *Gut, 5:*327, 1964.
274. Leger, L., Mouktar, M., and Lemaigre, G.: Pancreas et ulcere. Pancreas endocrine et diarrhee. Extension du syndrome de Zollinger-Ellison. *Act Hepatogastroent Hotel Dieu, 124:*55, 1964.
275. Lindner, A. E., Cohen, N., Berkowitz, J., *et al.:* A note on the oral dose of acetazolamide required to inhibit acid secretion in man. *Gastroenterology, 46:*273, 1964.
276. Malvy, P., Huard, M., Magre, J., *et al.:* Syndrome de Zollinger-Ellison avec diabete. *Mem Acad Chir (Paris), 90:*186, 1964.
277. Mandl, W.: Das Zollinger-Ellison syndrome. *Klin Med (Wien), 19:* 102, 1964.
278. McMahon, J. M., Justice, J., and Elliott, C. W.: An unusual case of the Zollinger-Ellison syndrome. *Am J Gastroent, 42:*271, 1964.
279. Newman, W. H., Bergen, F. D. O., and Roberts, D. C.: The Zollinger-Ellison syndrome. Recent experiences with two cases. *North Carolina Med, 25:*331, 1964.
280. Oberhelman, H. A., Jr., and Nelsen, T. S.: Surgical considerations in the management of ulcerogenic tumors of the pancreas and duodenum, *Am J Surg, 108:*132, 1964.
281. Oglesby, J. W., Mull, J. D., Humphries, A. L., Jr., *et al.:* Zollinger-Ellison syndrome in a nine-year-old boy. *Am J Surg, 108:*412, 1964.
282. Petrov, A. F.: Repeated and recurrent ulcer perforations in the stomach and duodenum. *Khirurgiia (Moskva), 40:*40, 1964.
283. Rapant, V.: Diagnostika nadoru pankreatu. *Prakt Lek, 44:*81, 1964.
284. Scobie, B. A., McGill, D. B., Priestly, J. T., *et al.:* Excluded gastric

antrum simulating the Zollinger-Ellison syndrome. *Gastroenterology, 47:*184, 1964.

285. Shafer, W. H.: Nonbeta islet-cell carcinoma of the pancreas presenting as diarrhea. Report of a case. *Ann Int Med, 61:*539, 1964.
286. Sircus, W.: Advances in gastroenterology. *Practitioner, 193:*509, 1964.
287. Sircus, W.: Evidence for a gastric secretagogue in the circulation and gastric juice of patients with the Zollinger-Ellison syndrome. *Lancet, 2:*671, 1964.
288. Sitenko, V. M., Samokhvalov, V. I., and Belousov, A. G.: The repeat recurrence of the peptic ulcer—The Zollinger-Ellison syndrome. *Vestn Khir Grekov, 93:*14, 1964.
289. State, D.: Gastrointestinal hormones in the production of peptic ulcer. *JAMA, 187:*410, 1964.
290. Tanner, N. C.: The surgical treatment of peptic ulcer. *Brit J Surg, 51:* 5, 1964.
291. Thayer, W. R., Jr.: Treatment of the intractable ulcer. *Mod Treat, 1:* 1499, 1964.
292. Veer, S. J. van der, Choufoer, J. C., Querido, A., *et al.:* Metastasizing islet cell tumor of the pancreas associated with hypoglycemia and carcinoid syndrome. *Lancet, 1:*1416, 1964.
293. Wegmann, R., Corcos, V., Albano, C., *et al.:* Histoenzymologie tumorale et gastrique d'une maladie de Zollinger-Ellison. *Sem Hop (Paris), 40:*1737, 1964.
294. Wegmann, T., Zollinger, H. U., and Markoff, N. G.: Zollinger-Ellison syndrom mit terminaler lethaler hypoglykamie. *Deutsch Med Wochenschr, 89:*2223, 1964.
295. Wruble, L. D.: The Zollinger-Ellison syndrome. *Memphis Med J, 39:* 45, 1964.
296. Wruble, L. D., Cole, G. W., Lessner, H. E., *et al.:* Evidence for the fundic origin of intrinsic factor. An in vivo study. *Ann Int Med, 60:*877, 1964.
297. Zollinger, R. M., and Grant, G. N.: Ulcerogenic tumor of the pancreas. *JAMA, 190:*181, 1964.

1965

298. Bank, S., Marks, I. N., Sealy, R., *et al.:* Malignant Zollinger-Ellison syndrome in a Bantu woman with a prolonged remission after gastric radiotherapy. *Gut, 6:*279, 1965.
299. Becker, V.: Das Zollinger-Ellison syndroms. Demonstration und deduktion. *Rev Int Hepat, 15:*509, 1965.
300. Becker, V.: Das Zollinger-Ellison syndrom. Paradigma der oberbaucheinheit. *Deutsch Ther, 16:*767, 1965.
301. Bonfils, S., Bader, J-P., Dubrasquet, M., *et al.:* Test biologiques explorant les facteurs gastrosecretagogues au cours du syndrome de Zollinger-Ellison. *Arch Mal App Dig, 54:*109, 1965.

302. Boutelier, P.: Un cas de syndrome de Zollinger-Ellison traite avec succes par gastrectomie totale. *Mem Acad Chir (Paris), 91:*257, 1965.
303. Bryant, J. G., and Smith, J. V.: Zollinger-Ellison syndrome with pancreatic islet cell hyperplasia. *Calif Med, 102:*49, 1965.
304. Cavallero, C., and Solcia, E.: Cytological and cytochemical aspects of islet pathology in the Zollinger-Ellison syndrome. *Rev Int Hepat, 15:*516, 1965.
305. DeMuth, W. E., Jr., and Smith, J. M.: Pancreatic biopsy in the diagnosis of Zollinger-Ellison syndrome. *Surgery, 57:*79, 1965.
306. Fontaine, R., Kieny, R., and Lang, G.: [Discovery by selective angiography of an ulcerogenic tumor of the pancreas of atypical symptomatology]. *Acad Chir, 91:*896, 1965.
307. Friesen, S. R.: Peptic ulcer. Endocrine factors in peptic ulceration, *J Kansas Med Soc, 66:*240, 1965.
308. Geokas, M. C., Chun, I. Y., Dinan, J. J., *et al.:* Islet cell carcinoma (Zollinger-Ellison syndrome) with fulminating adrenocortical hyperfunction and hypokalemia. *Canad Med Ass J, 93:*137, 1965.
309. Grann, V. R.: Islet cell neoplasms. *New York Med J, 65:*1976, 1965.
310. Herrington, J. L., Jr.: A teen-age boy with the Zollinger-Ellison syndrome presenting multiple ulcerations including perforation of a colonic ulcer. *Surgery, 58:*442, 1965.
311. Howe, C. T.: Ulcerogenic tumor of the pancreas. *Scot Med J, 10:*307, 1965.
312. Howe, C. T., Elliott, D. W., and Zollinger, R. M.: Total gastrectomy for the ulcerogenic tumor. In Ellison, E. H., Friesen, S. R., and Mulholland, J. H. (Eds.): *Current Surgical Management III.* Philadelphia: Saunders, 1965.
313. Hubens, A.: Role du foie dans le phase intestinale de la secretion acide de l'estomac. Etudie apres transpoition porto-cave chez le chien. *Rev Int Hepat, 15:*499, 1965.
314. Janser, J-C., Viville, C., Weill-Bousson, M., *et al.:* Le syndrome de Zollinger-Ellison. Localisations extopiques des tumeurs Langerhansiennes non hypoglycemiantes. A propos d'un cas opere et suivi depuis plus de 19 mois. *J Chir (Paris), 89:*346, 1965.
315. Kinnaird, D. W.: Hormone overproduction syndromes. Surgical considerations. *J Kentucky Med Ass, 63:*103, 1965.
316. Konaka, K., Matuoka, Y., Sibata, M., *et al.:* A powerful stimulant of gastric secretion extracted from the pancreas. *Kumamoto Med J, 18:* 234, 1965.
317. Lacerda, P.R.S., Dias, L. B., Schlee, J. C. C., *et al.:* Tumor ulcerogenico do duodeno. *Hospital (Rio), 68:*1013, 1965.
318. Lambling, A., Bonfils, S., Bader, J-P., *et al.:* Le pouvoir secretagogue gastrique des urines de l'homme (PSU). Interet clinique, en par-

ticulier dans le syndrome de Zollinger-Ellison. *Gastroent (Basel), 103*:152, 1965.

319. Law, D. H., Liddle, G. W., Scott, H. W., Jr., *et al.*: Ectopic production of multiple hormones (ACTH, MSH and gastrin) by a single malignant tumor. *New Eng J Med, 273*:292, 1965.
320. Lehner, A.: Zur behandlung des Zollinger-Ellison 'schen syndroms. *Rev Int Hepat, 15*:535, 1965.
321. Lowicki, E. M.: Gastrin and its surgical implications. *Surgery, 57*:602, 1965.
322. Melnyk, C. S., Krippaehne, W. W., Benson, J. A., Jr., *et al.*: Spontaneous remission of Zollinger-Ellison syndrome. *Arch Int Med, 115*:42, 1965.
323. Missakian, M., Carlson, H. C., and Huizenga, K. A.: Roentgenographic findings in Zollinger-Ellison syndrome. *Am J Roentgen, 94*:429, 1965.
324. Moucha, D.: Un cas de syndrome Zollinger-Ellison chez un garcon de 15 ans. *Bull Soc Chir (Paris), 55*:179, 1965.
325. Oberhelman, H. A., Jr.: Excision of ulcerogenic tumor. In Ellison, E. H., Friesen, S. R., and Mulholland, J. H. (Eds.): *Current Surgical Management III*, Philadelphia: Saunders, 1965.
326. Panchenkov, R. T.: [Gastric and duodenal ulcer in pancreatic adenomas]. *Klin Med (Moskva), 43*:88, 1965.
327. Parrish, J. A., and Rawlins, D. C.: Intestinal mucosa in the Zollinger-Ellison syndrome. *Gut, 6*:286, 1965.
328. Pernod, R., Hepp, J., Mercadier, M., *et al.*: Traitement chirurgical du syndrome de Zollinger-Ellison. A propos de 7 observations. *Ann Chir (Paris), 19*:1011, 1965.
329. Perrier, C. V.: The Zollinger-Ellison syndrome. Its place in the pathophysiology of gastric acid secretion and of its hormonal regulation. *Ergebn Inn Med Kinderheilk, 23*:89, 1965.
330. Potet, F. G., Bader, J-P., Martin, E., *et al.*: Etude histologique des ilots de Langerhans non tumoraux dans le syndrome de Zollinger-Ellison. Technique et resultats. *Arch Anat Path, 13*:206, 1965.
331. Preshaw, R. M., Cook, A. R., and Grossman, M. I.: Pancreatic secretion induced by stimulation of the pyloric gland area of the stomach. *Science, 148*:1347, 1965.
332. Provenale, L.: Interventi chirurgici su sindrome di Zollinger-Ellison. *Gezz Sanit, 36*:340, 1965.
333. Rapant, V., Dvoracek, C., Turek, K., *et al.*: Familial occurrence of the Zollinger-Ellison syndrome associated with diabetes. *Gastroent (Basel), 104*:289, 1965.
334. Reiswig, O. K., and Carter, R.: Polyendocrine adenomatosis with the Zollinger-Ellison syndrome. Successful treatment by total gastrectomy with a Lawrence Pouch. *Am Surg, 31*:695, 1965.

335. Rosenberg, R., and Janowitz, H. D.: The pancreas. IV. *Gastroenterology, 48:*350, 1965.
336. Ross, J. R., Warren, K. W., and Rudolph, N. E.: Zollinger-Ellison syndrome. Report of a case with a clinical appraisal of the syndrome. *Med Clin N Am, 50:*489, 1965.
337. Roufail, W. M., Boyette, G. T., Webster, P. D., *et al.:* Difficulties in the diagnosis of the Zollinger-Ellison syndrome. *Southern Med J, 58:*195, 1965.
338. Rubio, H. H., Pardo, R., Rivoira, J., *et al.:* Sindrome de Zollinger-Ellison. Actualizacion y referencia de un caso. *Presna Med Argent, 52:*2873, 1965.
339. Sacks, M. I.: Pancreatic tumor with repeated gastrointestinal hemorrhage and steatorrhea. *Israel J Med Sci, 1:*141, 1965.
340. San Juan, F., Treiger, M., Silvestre, W., *et al.:* Sindrome de Zollinger-Ellison. Apresentacao de um caso de adenoma de celulas nao-beta em pancreas heterotopico com ulceracao peptica duodeno-jejunal. *Hospital (Rio), 67:*1148, 1965.
341. Singleton, J. W., Kern, F., Jr., and Waddell, W. R.: Diarrhea and pancreatic islet cell tumor. Report of a case with a severe jejunal mucosal lesion. *Gastroenterology, 49:*197, 1965.
342. Sircus, W.: The Zollinger-Ellison syndrome. *Nurs Times, 61:*1719, 1965.
343. Sitenko, V. M., Samokhvalov, V. I., and Belousov, A. G.: [The repeat recurrence of the peptic ulcer. The Zollinger-Ellison syndrome]. *Vestn Khir Grekov, 93:*14, 1965.
344. Smith, R.: The Zollinger-Ellison syndrome. *Ann Roy Coll Surg (Eng), 37:*160, 1965.
345. Stewart, C. F.: Present status of surgery for peptic ulcer. *New York Med J, 65:*1996, 1965.
346. Wilson, H.: Zollinger-Ellison syndrome. *J Tenn Med Ass, 58:*341, 1965.
347. Wilson, S. D., and Ellison, E. H.: Total gastric resection in children with the Zollinger-Ellison syndrome. *Arch Surg, 91:*165, 1965.
348. Zollinger, R. M.: Ulcerogenic tumor of the pancreas. In Wells, C., and Kyle, J. (Eds.): *Scientific Foundations of Surgery.* New York: Elsevier, 176–179, 1965.
349. Zollinger, R. M., Taft, D. A., Endahl, G. L., *et al.:* Tumors of the isles of Langerhans. Ulcerogenic tumors. *Bull Soc Int Chir, 24:*343, 1965.

1966

350. Aoyagi, T., and Summerskill, W. H. J.: Gastric secretion with ulcerogenic islet cell tumor. Importance of basal acid output. *Arch Intern Med, 117:*667, 1966.
351. Bader, J. P., *et al.:* Gastro-secretogogue capacity of the urine in the Zollinger-Ellison syndrome. *Rev Int Hepat, 16:*723, 1966.

352. Bank, S., Marks, I. N., and Groll, A.: Gastric acid secretion in pancreatic disease. *Gastroenterology, 51*:649, 1966.
353. Becker, V.: Uber den Zollinger-Ellison mechanisms. *Klin Wochenschr, 44*:370–375, 1966.
354. Bondi, J. L.: Zollinger-Ellison syndrome. *Rev Sanid Milit Argent, 65*:45, 1966.
355. Britt, J. P.: Pedunculated islet cell tumor of the duodenum. *J Clin Path, 19*:272, 1966.
356. Christoforidis, A. J., and Nelson, S. W.: Radiological manifestations of ulcerogenic tumors of the pancreas. *JAMA, 198*:511, 1966.
357. Cook, H. B., and Lennard-Jones, J. E.: Effect of antisecretory drugs on gastric hypersecretion in endocrine-adenoma syndromes. *Lancet, 2*:247, 1966.
358. Dollinger, M. R., and Gardner, B.: Newer aspects of the carcinoid spectrum. (Collective review). *Surg Gynec Obstet, 122*:1335, 1966.
359. Dudek, W., and Beskid, M.: The Zollinger-Ellison syndrome in a patient with acromegaly. *Endokr Pol, 17*:341, 1966.
360. Gailitis, R. J.: The malignant carcinoid syndrome. Report of 5 cases. *Am J Dig Dis, 11*:630, 1966.
361. Gregory, R. A.: The isolation and chemistry of gastrin. *Gastroenterology, 51*:953, 1966.
362. Grossman, M. I.: Gastrin—reminiscence and speculation. *Am J Dig Dis, 11*:90, 1966.
363. Guida, P. M., Todd, J. E., Moore, S. W., *et al.*: Zollinger-Ellison syndrome with interesting variations. Report of 12 cases including one of carcinoid of the duodenum. *Am J Surg, 112*:807, 1966.
364. Hakoda, M., Matsumoto, H., and Nakajio, S.: Zollinger-Ellison syndrome. *Surg Ther (Osaka), 15*:408, 1966.
365. Hellmans, N., DeBoer, W. G. R. M., and Julius, J.: Persistent ulcer and Zollinger-Ellison syndrome. *Nederl T Geneesk, 110*:298, 1966.
366. Huslarova, A., Niederle, B., and Rachenberg, M.: Zollingeruv-Ellisonuv syndrom a frustni symptomatologii. *Sborn Lek, 68*:303, 1966.
367. Iwasa, H., Koshibu, K., Okamoto, Y., *et al.*: Zollinger-Ellison syndrome. *Surg Ther (Osaka), 15*:408, 1966.
368. Kalashnikov, S. A.: The structure of tumors in the Zollinger-Ellison syndrome. *Vop Onkol, 12*:10, 1966.
369. Kirsner, J. B.: Peptic ulcer—a review of the literature for 1965. *Gastroenterology, 51*:403, 1966.
370. Konturek, S., and Grossman, M. I.: Acid response to gastrin and related peptides. *Gastroenterology, 50*:650, 1966.
371. Ludin, H., Enderlin, F., Fahrlander, H. J., *et al.*: Failure to diagnose

Zollinger-Ellison syndrome by pancreatic arteriography. *Brit J Radiol, 39:*494, 1966.
372. Ludin, H., Fahrlander, H. J., and Renggli, I.: Zur darstellung von Karzinoid-Lebermetastasen mittels visceraler arteriographie. *Schweiz Med Wochenschr, 96:*1642, 1966.
373. McGavran, M. H., Unger, R. H., Recant, L., *et al.:* A glucagon-secreting-alpha cell carcinoma of the pancreas. *New Eng J Med, 274:*1408, 1966.
374. Merdinger, I.: Fatal intestinal hemorrhage and multiple endocrine adenomata. *Dapim Refuiim (Tel-Aviv), 24:*457, 1966.
375. Murphy, D. L., Goldstein, H., Boyle, J. D., *et al.:* Hypercalcemia and gastric secretion in man. *J App Physiol, 21:*5:1607, 1966.
376. Oda, M., Matsuoka, T., Miyashita, H., *et al.:* A case of Zollinger-Ellison syndrome. *J Jap Soc Intern Med, 55:*886, 1966.
377. Outz, L., Gaines, C. D., Donald, J. M., Jr., *et al.:* Recurrent peptic ulceration associated with pancreatic lesions: Zollinger-Ellison syndrome case report. *Amer Surg, 32:*57, 1966.
378. Pampari, D., and Bordi, C.: Anatomic-clinical study on a case of the Zollinger-Ellison syndrome. *Minerva Chir, 21:*15, 1966.
379. Polileux, F., and Mouktar, M.: Non-beta cell insular tumors of the duodenum or Zollinger-Ellison duodenal tumors. *Act Hepatogastroent Hotel Dieu,* July-Sept., 1966.
380. Polacek, M. A., and Ellison, E. H.: Gastric acid secretion and parietal cell mass in the stomach of a newborn infant. *Am J Surg, 111:*777, 1966.
381. Polacek, M. A., and Ellison, E. H.: Parietal cell mass and gastric secretion in the Zollinger-Ellison syndrome. *Surgery, 60:*606, 1966.
382. Ragins, H., and Braylan, R. C.: Zollinger-Ellison tumor associated with a malabsorption syndrome. With abdominal distention resembling large bowel obstruction. *Am J Surg, 112:*441, 1966.
383. Schulte, W. J., and Ellison, E. H.: Effect of total gastrectomy on growth in puppies. *Am J Surg, 111:*782, 1966.
384. Scobie, B. A., and Beetham, D. T.: Zollinger-Ellison syndrome due to duodenal ectopic islet cell tumor. *New Zeal Med J, 65:*979, 1966.
385. Tuncel, S., Degerli, U., and Pars, B.: Zollinger-Ellison sendromu. *Turk Tip Cem Mec, 32:*630, 1966.
386. Wall, G., Duque, J., and O'Brien, T.: Diagnosis of the Zollinger-Ellison syndrome in a patient with subtotal gastrectomy. *Virginia Med Monthly, 93:*575, 1966.
387. Wormsley, K. G., Mahoney, M. P., and Margaret, N. G.: Effect of a gastrin-like pentapeptide on stomach and pancreas. *Lancet, 1:* 994, 1966.
388. Zaterka, S., and Grossman, M. I.: The effect of gastrin and histamine on secretion of bile. *Gastroenterology, 50:*500, 1966.

389. Zollinger, R. M.: Relationship of the pancreas and other endocrine glands to peptic ulcer. *Rev Int Hepat, 16:*715, 1966.
390. Zollinger, R. M.: Ulcerogenic tumors of the pancreas. *Rev Int Hepat, 16:*649, 1966.
391. Zollinger, R. M., Endahl, G., Moore, F. T., *et al.:* Ulcerogenic tumors of the pancreas. *The Cancer Bulletin, 28:*79, Houston: The Medical Arts Publishing Foundation, February, 1966.
392. Zollinger, R. M., Moore, F. T., Endahl, G. L., *et al.:* Ulcerogenic tumor of the pancreas. *J Czech Gastro Nut, 20:*443, 1966.

1967

393. Abernethy, R. J., Gillespie, I. E., Lawrie, J. H., *et al.:* Pentagastrin as a stimulant of maximal acid response in man. A multicentre pilot study. *Lancet, 1:*291, 1967.
394. Andersson, S. and Nilsson, G.: Duodenal inhibition of gastric secretion. In Shnitka, T. K., Gilbert, J. A. L. and Harrison, R. C. (Eds.): *Gastric Secretion: Mechanisms and Control.* Long Island: Pergamon Press, 1967.
395. Anokhina, L. I.: Clinical picture of ulcerogenic adenoma of the pancreas (Zollinger-Ellison syndrome). *Probl Endokr (Moskva), 13:* 21, 1967.
396. Bader, J. P., Bonfils, S., Ferrier, J. P., *et al.:* The Zollinger-Ellison syndrome. A clinical, biological and anatomical study of 10 observations. *Presse Med, 53:*2709, 1967.
397. Bader, J. P., Bonfils, S., and Lambling, A.: Insular adenoma with alpha cells. Clinical and biologic data. *Acta Hepatogastroent Hotel Dieu,* 1967.
398. Balazs, M., Haas, P., and Herczeg, T.: Ulcerogenic islet cell adenoma in the duodenum. Zollinger-Ellison syndrome. *Orv Hetil, 108:*1600, 1967.
399. Bank, S., Marks, I. N., Louw, J. H., *et al.:* The augmented histamine test. A review of 5,364 tests. *Recent Adv Gastroent, 1:*399, 1967.
400. Bennet, J.: Apropos of a case of Zollinger-Ellison syndrome. Act. *Hepatogastroent Hotel Dieu,* 1967.
401. Bergoz, R., and Rohner, A.: Zollinger-Ellison syndrome of the diarrhea form. On the basis of one case. *Schweiz Med Wochenschr, 97:*413, 1967.
402. Berson, S. A., and Yalow, R. S.: Radioimmunoassays of peptide hormones in plasma. *New Eng J Med, 277:*640, 1967.
403. Borovyi, E. M., and Bas, V. M.: 3-Stage resection of the stomach for Zollinger-Ellison syndrome. *Khirurgiia (Moskva), 43:*122, 1967.
404. Brown, G. E., Faustina, G. E., and Orloff, M. J.: Humoral mediation of the intestinal phase of gastric secretion. *Surg Forum, 18:*298, 1967.
405. Burge, H.: Pathophysiological problems of vagotomy in ulcer disease. *Zbl Chir, 92:*1233, 1967.

406. Buckley, R. E.: Induction of hyperglycaemia as treatment for peptic ulcers. *Lancet, 11*:497, 1967.
407. Castell, D. I., Sparks, H. A., and Johnson, R. B.: The importance of fluoroscopic tube placement during gastric analysis. *Am J Dig Dis, 12*:26, 1967.
408. Cavallero, C., Solcia, E., and Sampietro, R.: Cytology of islet tumors and hyperplasias associated with the Zollinger-Ellison syndrome. *Gut, 8*:172, 1967.
409. Cavallero, C., Solcia, E., Vassallo, G., *et al.*: Morpho-biologic aspects of Zollinger-Ellison syndrome. *Arch Ital Mal Appar Dig, 34*:53, 1967.
410. Church, R. E., and Crane, W. A. J.: A cutaneous syndrome associated with islet-cell carcinoma of the pancreas. *Brit J Derm, 79*:284, 1967.
411. Clemett, A. R.: Arteriographic demonstration of pancreatic tumor in the Zollinger-Ellison syndrome. *Radiology, 88*:32, 1967.
412. Connell, A. M., and Logan, C. J. H.: The role of gastrin in gastroileocolic responses. *Am J Dig Dis, 12*:227, 1967.
413. DaCruz, G. M., Gardner, J. D., and Peskin, G. W.: Influence of gastrointestinal tumors on intestinal absorption. *Surg Forum, 18*: 336, 1967.
414. Demling, L.: Clinical picture and therapy of enteritis. *Wien Klin Wochenschr, 79*:597, 1967.
415. Ellison, E. H., and Wilson, S. D.: The Zollinger-Ellison syndrome updated. *Surg Clin N Am, 47*:1115, 1967.
416. Ellison, E. H., and Wilson, S. D.: Ulcerogenic tumor of the pancreas. *Prog Clin Cancer, 3*:225, 1967.
417. Ermini, M., and Carboni, M.: Possibilities of experimental reproduction of Zollinger-Ellison syndrome. *Arch Ital Mal Appar Dig, 34*:81, 1967.
418. Fiorini, E., Fratton, A., Marabini, A., *et al.*: On a case of Zollinger-Ellison syndrome followed during 6 years. Contribution to the interpretation of scintigraphy in operated pancreas. *Arch Ital Mal Appar Dig, 34*:86, 1967.
419. Friesen, S. R.: Effect of total gastrectomy on the Zollinger-Ellison tumor: Observations by second-look procedures. *Surgery, 62*:609, 1967.
420. Garcia, E. L., Guedes, J. R., Berastequi, V. N., *et al.*: Remarks on a case of the Zollinger-Ellison syndrome. *Rev Clin Esp, 304,* 1967.
421. Gardner, J. D., Peskin, G. W., Cerda, J. J., *et al.*: Alterations of in vitro fluid and electrolyte absorption by gastrointestinal hormones. *Am J Surg, 113*:57, 1967.
422. Gelder, A. van, Houten, H. van, Ronnen, J. R. von, *et al.*: Diarrhea and gastric acid secretion and the Zollinger-Ellison syndrome. *Nederl T Geneesk, 111*:15, 1967.

423. Gobbel, W. G., Jr., and Adkins, R. B.: Production of duodenal ulcers by exogenous gastrin. An experimental model. *Am J Surg, 113:* 183, 1967.
424. Gregory, R. A., Grossman, M. I., Tracy, H. J., *et al.:* Nature of the gastric secretagogue in Zollinger-Ellison tumours. *Lancet, 11:*543, 1967.
425. Grossman, M. I.: A prize unclaimed. *Gastroenterology, 52:*918, 1967.
426. Grossman, M. I.: Some aspects of gastric secretion. *Gastroenterology, 52:*882, 1967.
427. Gudas, P. P., Jr., Haberman, G. G., and Belcher, H. V.: Cholecytocolonic fistula. *Arch Surg, 95:*228, 1967.
428. Hardy, J. D.: Complications of gastric resection. In Artz, C. P., and Hardy, J. D. (Eds.): *Complications in Surgery and Their Management,* 2nd ed. Philadelphia, Saunders, 446, 1967.
429. Haugen, O. A.: Strom-Zollinger-Ellison syndrom. *Nord Med, 78:*1094, 1967.
430. Helbock, H., Davidson, W. D., Lemmi, C. A. E., *et al.:* Effect of a gastrin-like pentapeptide on the flux of ions across the isolated gastric mucosa of the bullfrog. *Surg Forum, 18:*319, 1967.
431. Hiatt, R. B., Goodman, I., and Alavi, A.: Hormonal control of intestinal motility. *Ann Surg, 166:*704, 1967.
432. Hurvitz, R. J., Hurvitz, J. S., and Morgenstern, L.: In vivo staining of the parathyroid glands and pancreas. *Arch Surg, 95:*274, 1967.
433. Irvine, W. J., McLoughlin, G. P., Stewart, A. G., *et al.:* Appraisal of the Application of ^{99m} TC in the assessment of gastric function. *Lancet, 2:*648, 1967.
434. Jarrett, R. J., and Cohen, N. M.: Intestinal hormones and plasma-insulin. *Lancet, 2:*861, 1967.
435. Jesseph, J. E., Moore, F. T., Endahl, G. L., *et al.:* Peptic ulceration and enteritis. A differential diagnosis. *Am J Surg, 113:*188, 1967.
436. Johnson, G. J., Summerskill, W. H. J., Anderson, V. E., *et al.:* Clinical and genetic investigation of a large kindred with multiple endocrine adenomatosis. *New Eng J Med, 277:*1379, 1967.
437. Johnston, D., and Jepson, K.: Use of pentagastrin in a test of gastric acid secretion. *Lancet, 2:*585, 1967.
438. Kay, A. W.: An evaluation of gastric acid secretion tests. *Gastroenterology, 53:*834, 1967.
439. Keel, H. J.: Gastric juice analysis. *Schweiz Med Wachenschr, 97:*1079, 1967.
440. Keel, H. J., and Roth, J. L.: Islet cell tumors not producing insulin. *Schweitz Med Wochenschr, 97:*1399, 1967.
441. Kerr, G. D., and Smith, R.: Hypercalcemia and gastric hypersecretion in the familial endocrine-adenoma syndrome. *Lancet, 1:*1074, 1967.
442. Klepping, C., Cabanne, F., and Aupecle, P.: Nonsecretory nesidioblas-

toma of ectopic localization (duodenal). *Acta Hepatógastroent Hotel Dieu,* 1967.

443. Kusakcioglu, O., and Heffernan, E.: Zollinger-Ellison syndrome. Amer *J Gastroent, 48:*110, 1967.
444. Laszlo, A., and Ormos, J.: Simultaneous occurrence of Zollinger-Ellison syndrome and pancreatic cystadenoma. *Orv Hetil, 108:*1603, 1967.
445. Liu, D. H., Crastnopol, P., and Phillips, W.: Perforation of a gastrojejunal ulcer into the pericardium. Complications of Wermer's disease (Zollinger-Ellison syndrome). *Arch Surg, 94:*294, 1967.
446. Logan, C. J. H.: Gastrin as an intestinal activator. *Brit J Surg, 54,* 297, 1967.
447. Lynch, H. T.: *Hereditary Factors in Carcinoma.* New York, Springer-Verlag, 26, 1967.
448. Maiat, V. S. and Keshisheva, A. A.: Zollinger-Ellison syndrome. *Khirurgi:a (Moskva), 43:*3, 1967.
449. Martin, E. D., and Potet, F.: Histopathology of the Zollinger-Ellison syndrome. *Ac:a Hepatógastro Hotel Dieu,* 1967.
450. McGuigan, J. E.: Antibodies to the carboxyl-terminal tetrapeptide of gastrin. *Gastroenterology, xx:* 697, 1967.
451. McPhedran, N. T. *et al.:* The nature and source of a gastric secretagogue. *Arch Surg, 95:*606, 1967.
452. Mlinaric, I., and Urbanke, A.: Cystic insular adenoma of the pancreas associated with Zollinger-Ellison syndrome. *Rad Med Fak Zagreb, 15:*25, 1967.
453. Moore, F. T., *et al.:* Diagnosis of ulcerogenic tumor of the pancreas by bioassay. *Amer J Surg, 113:*735, 1967.
454. Murata, I., and Hirono, T.: Clinical and pathological observations of pancreas induced ulcer. Proc. 67th Annual Congress of Japan Surgical Society, Nagoya, March 30-31, pp. 9, 1967.
455. Ottenjann, R., Gall, F., and Elster, K.: Tumor-like hyperplasia of the gastric mucosa of the Zollinger-Ellison syndrome. *Deutsch Med Wochenschr, 92:*1538, 1967.
456. Paloyan, D., *et al.:* Gastric hypersecretion induced by parathyroidectomy in the dog. *Surg Forum, 18:*347, 1967.
457. Panchenkov, R. T., and Datsenko, V. S.: The Zollinger-Ellison syndrome. *Klin Med (Moskva), 45:*76, 1967.
458. Passaro, E., Jr., and Gordon, H. E.: Gastric secretory tests. Pro and con. *Am J Surg, 114:*333, 1967.
459. Pencev, J.: Gastroduenalni vred pri rakovine prostaty obmena Zollingerova-Ellisonova syndromu. *Vnitrni Lek, 13:*760, 1967.
460. Perrotin, J., and Hautefeuille, P.: Surgical treatment of the Zollinger-Ellison syndrome. *Acta Hepatógastro Hotel Dieu,* 1967.
461. Pissidis, G. A., and Clark, C. G.: An improved technique of perfusion of the stomach for the study of gastric secretion in the rat. *Gut, 8:*196, 1967.

462. Ringler, W., and Wedell, J.: Intraoperative and postoperative complications in the surgical management for peptic ulcer of the jejunum. *Zbl Chir, 92:*2367, 1967.
463. Rosenlund, M. L.: The Zollinger-Ellison syndrome in children. A review. *Am J Med Sci, 254:*134, 1967.
464. Roux, M.: The Zollinger-Ellison syndrome. *Cahiers college Med hop (Paris), 8:*2, 1967.
465. Ruppert, R. D., Greenberger, N. J., Beman, F. M., *et al.:* Gastric secretion in ulcerogenic tumors of the pancreas. *Ann Intern Med, 67:*808, 1967.
466. Rydgier, J., Wiechno, W., Kobuszewska-Faryna, M., *et al.:* A case of the Zollinger-Ellison syndrome. *Pol Arch Med Wewnet, 38:*365, 1967.
467. Saegesser, M.: Surgical aspects of ulcer disease. *Praxis, 56:*440, 1967.
468. Sapkas, V. A., Litsios, B.: Fin fall von Zollinger-Ellison syndrom. *Zb1 Chir, 18,* 1967.
469. Sapkas, A., and Litsios, B.: One case of Zollinger-Ellison syndrome. *Zb1 Chir,* 92:648, 1967.
470. Schneider, D. R., Endahl, G. L., Dodd, M. C., *et al.:* Gastrin antibodies: Induction, demonstration, and specificity. *Science, 156:*391, 1967.
471. Silen, W.: Advances in gastric physiology. *New Eng J Med, 277:*864, 1967.
472. Smallwood, R. A.: Effect of intravenous calcium administration on gastric secretion of acid and pepsin in man. *Gut, 8:*592, 1967.
473. Stefanini, P.: Clinical aspects of Zollinger-Ellison syndrome. *Arch Ital Mal Appar Dig, 34:*76, 1967.
474. Stiel, J. N., Mitchell, C. A., Radcliff, F. J., *et al.:* Hypercalcemia in patients with peptic ulceration receiving large doses of calcium carbonate. *Gastroenterology, 53:*900, 1967.
475. Stremple, J. F., Abramoff, P., van Oss, J. C., *et al.:* Antibodies to synthetic human gastrin I. *Lancet, 2:*1180, 1967.
476. Thiery, J.-P., and Bader, J. P.: Electron microscope study of islet cell tumors with alpha cells in the Zollinger-Ellison syndrome. *Acta Hepat Hotel Dieu,* 1967.
477. Toker, C.: Some observations on the ultrastructure of a malignant islet cell tumor associated with duodenal ulceration and severe diarrhea. *J Ultrastruct Res, 19:*522, 1967.
478. Van Gelden, A., Van Houten, H., Von Ronnen, J. R., *et al.:* Diarrhea and stomach juice production in the Zollinger-Ellison syndrome. *Nederl T Geneesk, 111:*15, 1967.
479. Vayre, P., Terris, G., Hureau, J., *et al.:* Multiple ulcers of the second duodenum and acute perforation accident. Pancreatic tumor. Mesenteric and ganglioner metastases. *J Chir (Paris), 93:*351, 1967.
480. Vogel, R. M., Weinstein, L. D., Herskovic, T., and *et al.:* Mechanisms

of steatorrhea in the Zollinger-Ellison syndrome. *Ann Intern Med, 67:816,* 1967.

481. Weichert, R., Reed, R., and Creech, O., Jr.: Carcinoid-islet cell tumors of the duodenum. *Ann Surg, 165:*660, 1967.
482. Weinshelbaum, E. I., *et al.:* A secretory influence of gastric enterochromaffin cells. *Surg Forum, 18:*342, 1967.
483. Wermer, P.: The Diagnosis of Polyadenomatosis of endocrine glands. *Radiol Clin N Am, 5:*349, 1967.
484. Wilken, B. J., Hunt, D. G., Lowe, C. F., *et al.:* Sensitivity, range, and reliability of a method for the bioassay of gastrin. *J Surg Res, 9:*551, 1967.
485. Williams, L. F., Jr.: Intestinal electrolyte transport. *Surg Forum, 18:*321, 1967.
486. Winship, D. H., and Ellison, E. H.: Variability of gastric secretion in patients with and without the Zollinger-Ellison syndrome. *Lancet, 1:*1128, 1967.
487. Zenker, R., and Grabiger, A.: New views of the surgery of endocrine diseases. *Bruns Beitr Klin Chir, 214:*41, 1967.
488. Zollinger, R. M.: Hormones affecting gastric secretion. *Pacific Med Surg, 83:*1967.
489. Zollinger, R. M.: Reflections on the ulcerogenic syndrome. *Am Surg, 33:*610, 1967.
490. Zollinger, R. M.: Ulcerogenic tumor of the pancreas. In Wells, C., and Kyle, J. (Eds.): *Scientific Foundations of Surgery.* New York: Elsevier, 176, 1967.

1968

491. Adair, R. K., and Wlodek, G. K.: Ionic changes in pavlov pouches after insulin hypoglycemia, gastrin and pentagastrin. *Arch Surg, 97:*423, 1968.
492. Adams, J.: The clinical and metabolic consequences of total gastrectomy II. Anaemia, metabolism of iron, vitamin B-12 and folic acid. *Scand J Gastroent, 3:*145, 1968.
493. Adams, J.: The clinical and metabolic consequences of total gastrectomy III. Notes on metabolic functions, deficiency states, changes in intestinal histology and radiology. *Scand J Gastroent, 3:*152, 1968.
494. Assan, R., Tohobroutsky, G., and Rosselin, G.: A case of hypoglycemic beta-langerhansian adenoma and secreting parathyroidian adenoma-polyadenomatosis. *Presse Med, 76:*2259, 1968.
495. Bedacht, R., and Rueff, F. L.: Insulin producing and non-insulin producing pancreatic tumors with endocrine disease features. *Munchen Med Wochenschr, 110:*446, 1968.
496. Bouchier, I. A.: Cancer of the pancreas. *Brit Med J, 3:*169, 1968.

497. Brown, R. E., and Still, W. J.: Nesidioblastosis and the Zollinger-Ellison syndrome. *Am J Dig Dis, 13:*656, 1968.
498. Caridis, D. T., Porter, J. F., and Smith, G.: Detection of histamine in venous blood from the stomach during acid secretion evoked by intravenous pentagastrin. *Lancet, 1:*1281, 1968.
499. Clayman, C. B., Palmer, W. L., and Kirsner, J. B.: Gastric irradiation in the treatment of peptic ulcer. *Gastroenterology, 55:*403, 1968.
500. Cooke, A. R.: Observations on the effect of diversion of acid from the duodenum in response to gastrin and histamine. *Gastroenterology, 55:*268, 1968.
501. Copeland, E. M., Miller, L. D., and Smith, G. P.: The complex nature of small bowel control of gastric secretion. *Ann Surg, 168:*36, 1968.
502. Dimbiloglu, M. E., Appert, H. E., Howard, J. M., *et al.:* The relative tolerance of the dog to intravenous infusions of pancreatic juice. *Surgery, 64:*805, 1968.
503. Doll, R., Langman, M. J. S., and Shawdon, H. H.: Treatment of gastric ulcer with estrogens. *Gut, 9:*46, 1968.
504. Emas, S., and Grossman, M. I.: Acid responses to graded doses of histamine and gastrin in heidenhain pouch cats. *Gastroenterology, 55:*72, 1968.
505. Emas, S., Billings, A., and Grossman, M. I.: Effects of gastrin and pentagastrin on gastric and pancreatic secretion in dogs. *Scand J Gastroent, 3:*234, 1968.
506. Friesen, S. R.: A gastric factor in the pathogenesis of the Zollinger-Ellison syndrome. *Ann Surg, 168:*483, 1968.
507. Galmarini, O. V.: Current approach to Zollinger-Ellison's syndrome. *Prensa Med Argent, 55:*1265, 1968.
508. Gillespie, I. E.: The surgical treatment of peptic ulcer. *Postgrad Med J, 44:*608, 1968.
509. Gordon, S. J., Haro, E. N., Paes, I. C., *et al.:* Studies of malabsorption and calcium excretion induced by neomycin sulfate. Effect on intestinal site, bile salt and pancreatic enzymes. *JAMA 204:*129, 1968.
510. Grafe, W. R., Loehr, W., and Thorbjarnarson, B.: Gastroenterostomy and vagotomy in the treatment of duodenal ulcer disease. *Ann Surg, 168:*966, 1968.
511. Henrikksen, F. W.: Effect of pancreozymin of the canine pancreatic secretion of fluid and bicarbonate. *Scand J Gastroent, 3:*637, 1968.
512. Hillman, H. S.: Postgastrectomy nutrition. *Gut, 9:*576, 1968.
513. Hirschowitz, B. I.: Apparent kinetics of histamine dose-responsive gastric water and electrolyte secretion in the dog. *Gastroenterology, 54:*514, 1968.
514. Hubel, K. A.: The ins and outs of bicarbonate in the alimentary tract. *Gastroenterology, 54:*647, 1968.

515. Huberman, E. D., Berra, J. L., and Santana, M. A.: Zollinger-Ellison syndrome. Presentation of a case. *Rev Clin Esp, 111:*431, 1968.
516. Jepson, K., and Johnston, D.: Effect of vagotomy on human gastric acid secretion stimulated by gastrin pentapeptide and by histalog. *Gastroenterology, 55:*665, 1968.
517. Kauffman, H. J., and Spiro, H. M.: Estrogens and gastric secretion. *Gastroenterology, 54:*913, 1968.
518. Kim, Y. S., and Spritz, N.: Hydroxy acid excretion in steatorrhea of pancreatic and nonpancreatic origin. *New Eng J Med, 279:*1424, 1968.
519. Kirk, R. M.: Site and localization of duodenal ulcers: a study at operation. *Gut, 9:*414, 1968.
520. Konturek, S. J.: The effect of secretin on gastric acid secretion and peptic ulcers induced by pentagastrin in cats with intact or resected duodenum. *Am J Dig Dis, 13:*874, 1968.
521. Kraft, A. R., Tompkins, R. K., Endahl, G. L., *et al.:* Hydrelatic effect of brocresine on the exocrine pancreas. *Clin Res, 16:*448, 1968.
522. Lee, J. S., and Duncan, K. M.: Lymphatic and venous transport of water from rat jejunum: a vascular perfusion study. *Gastroenterology, 54:*559, 1968.
523. Lewin, M., and Bonfils, S.: Statistic evaluation of the correlation of acid-pepsin (K25) in human gastric juice in health and disease. *Rev Franc Etud Clin Biol, 13:*780, 1968.
524. Lotz, M., Zisman, E., *et al.:* Evidence for a phosphorus-depletion syndrome in man. *New Eng J Med, 278:*409, 1968.
525. Maiorov, V. M., Ponomarenko, V. N., and Revzis, M. G.: On ulcers of the gastrointestinal tract in ulcerogenic adenoma of the pancreas. *Klin Med (Moskva), 46:*110, 1968.
526. Mannix, H., Jr., and Loehr, W. J.: Unusual aspects of hyperparathyroidism. *Surg Gynec Obstet, 126:*347, 1968.
527. Mansford, K. R. L., and Opie, L.: Comparison of metabolic abnormalities in diabetes mellitus induced by streptozotocin or by alloxan. *Lancet, 1:*670, 1968.
528. McGuigan, J. E., and Trudeau, W. L.: Immunochemical measurement of elevated levels of gastrin in the serum of patients with pancreatic tumors of the Zollinger-Ellison variety. *New Eng J Med, 278 (24):*1308, 1968.
529. McIlrath, D. C.: Gastroenterology at the surgical forum in 1967. A review. *Gastroenterology, 54:*667, 1968.
530. Melmed, R. N., Agnew, J. E., and Bouchier, I. A.: The normal and abnormal pancreatic scan. *Quart J Med, 37:*607, 1968.
531. Menguy, R., and Desbaillets, L.: The gastric mucous barrier: influence of protein-bound carbohydrate in mucus on the rate of proteolysis of gastric mucus. *Ann Surg, 168:*475, 1968.

532. Merz, T., El-Mahdi, A. M., and Prempree, T.: Unusual chromosomes and malignant disease. *Lancet, 1:*337, 1968.
533. Moore, E. W., and Makhlouf, G. M.: Calcium in normal human gastric juice, a four-component model with speculation on the relation of calcium to pepsin secretion. *Gastroenterology, 55:*465, 1968.
534. Moore, F. T., Nadler, S. H., Radefeld, D. A., *et al.:* Prolonged remission of diarrhea due to non-beta islet cell tumors of the pancreas by radiotherapy. *Am J Surg, 115:*854, 1968.
535. Myszka, S., Oleszak, H., and Jedrzejczyk, W.: Clinical picture and pathologic anatomical changes in the Ellison-Zollinger syndrome. *Pol Przegl Chir, 40:*266, 1968.
536. Nakamura, M., Nakajima, S., and Magee, D. F.: Action of pancreozymin preparations on gastric acid secretion. *Gut, 9:*405, 1968.
537. Nance, F. C., and Thomas, M. A.: Diagnosis and treatment of the Zollinger-Ellison syndrome. *J Louisiana Med Soc, 120:*91, 1968.
538. Nicoloff, D. M.: Indomethacin. Effect on gastric secretion, parietal cell population and ulcer provocation in the dog. *Arch Surg, 97:* 809, 1968.
539. Ottenjann, R., and Peters, H.: Gastric secretion analysis in the Zollinger-Ellison syndrome. *Klin Wochenschr, 46:*870, 1968.
540. Pascal, J. P., Sannou, N., and Ribet, A.: Exploration of pancreatic exocrine function by continuous infusion of secretin. *Amer J Dig Dis, 13:*213, 1968.
541. Porta, G. C., and D'Alonzo, U.: A case of association of pancreatic adenoma and double duodenal ulcer. *Osped Ital Chir, 19:*329, 1968.
542. Rienhoff, W. F., Jr., Rienhoff, W. F., III, Brawley, R. K., *et al.:* The surgical treatment of hyperparathyroidism. *Ann Surg, 168:*1061, 1968.
543. Roselli, A.: Zollinger-Ellison syndrome. Current concepts of its pathology. *Hospital (Rio), 73:*1411, 1968.
544. Ryss, S., and Ryss, E.: Modern concept of etiology and pathogenesis of peptic ulcer. Disorders of the regulating mechanisms. *Scand J Gastroent, 3:*513, 1968.
545. Samokhvalov, V. I., and Kalashnikov, S. A.: Zollinger-Ellison syndrome during malignant degeneration of adenomas of the pancreas. *Vop Onkol, 14:*24, 1968.
546. Schuck, M., Santillani, M., Wise, L., *et al.:* Studies on the inhibition of gastric secretion by the small intestine. *Surg Gynec Obstet, 127:* 1295, 1968.
547. Self, J. B.: A gastric reconstruction. *Brit J Surg, 55:*602, 1968.
548. Silber, W.: Pressure studies in the diagnosis of esophageal disease. *Am J Dig Dis, 13:*356, 1968.
549. Skala, I., Krondl, A., Vulterinova, M., *et al.:* Composition of feces in

steatorrhea of different etiology: Mutual relationship between the volume of feces, water, dry matter, nitrogen and fat content. *Am J Dig Dis, 13:*204, 1968.
550. Soustelle, J., Chevillard, R., Bertocchi, R., *et al.:* Multiple and recurrent perforations after gastrectomy for ulcer—Zollinger-Ellison syndrome. *Lyon Chir, 64:*804, 1968.
551. Thompson, J. C., Davidson, W. D., Patton, J. J., *et al.:* Histamine stimulation of gastric pepsin secretion in the dog. *Arch Surg, 97:* 805, 1968.
552. Vagne, M., and Grossman, M. I.: Cholecystokinetic potency of gastrointestinal hormones and related peptides. *Am J Physiol, 215:*881, 1968.
553. Vance, J. E., Kitabchi, A. E., and Buchanan, K. D.: Hypersecretion of insulin, glucagon, and gastrin in a kindred with multiple adenomatosis. *Diabetes, 17:*299, 1968.
554. Way, L., Goldman, L., and Dunphy, J. E.: Zollinger-Ellison syndrome. An analysis of twenty-five cases. *Am J Surg, 116:*293, 1968.
555. Wiechno, W., Poltorak, J. L., and Zawadzki, J. S.: Surgical management in Zollinger-Ellison syndrome. *Wiad Lek, 21:*1539, 1968.
556. Wilson, S. D., Mathison, J. A., Schulte, W. J., *et al.:* The role of bioassay in the diagnosis of ulcerogenic tumors. *Arch Surg, 97:*437, 1968.
557. Wormsley, K. G.: Gastric response to secretin and pancreozymin in man. *Scand J Gastroent, 3:*632, 1968.
558. Wormsley, K. G.: Pentagastrin snuff. A new means of stimulating gastric secretion. *Lancet, 1:*57, 1968.
559. Zboralske, F. F., and Amberg, J. R.: Detection of the Zollinger-Ellison syndrome—The radiologist-s responsibility. *Am J Roentgen, 104:* 529, 1968.
560. Zollinger, R. M., and Moore, F. T.: Zollinger-Ellison syndrome comes of age. Recognition of the complete clinical spectrum and its management. *JAMA 204:*361, 1968.

1969

561. *Abstract of* Zollinger, R. M., and Moore, F. T.: Zollinger-Ellison syndrome. *Rev Clin Esp, 112:*211, 1969.
562. Alfidi, R. J., Skillern, P. G., and Crile, G., Jr.: Arteriographic manifestations of the Zollinger-Ellison syndrome. Report of a case. *Cleve Clin Quart, 36:*41, 1969.
563. Antic, R., Grant, A. K., and Meadows, S. R.: Zollinger-Ellison syndrome—A report of three cases. *Aust Ann Med, 18:*277, 1969.
564. Arzua, E., Obregon, J. L., Tanago, J. G., *et al.:* Zollinger-Ellison syndrome. *Rev Clin Esp, 115:*335, 1969.
565. Ayas, E., Lamagna, C., Herrera, R., *et al.:* Zollinger-Ellison syndrome,

ulcerogenic tumors of the pancreas. *Prensa Med Argent, 56:*778, 1969.

566. Betaneli, A. M., and Kantariia, V. V.: The casuistics of the Zollinger-Ellison syndrome. *Khirurgiia (Moskva), 45:*68, 1969.

567. Blair, E. L., Falkmer, S., Hellerstrom, C., *et al.*: Investigation of gastrin activity in pancreatic islet tissue. *Acta Path Microbiol Scand, 75:* 583, 1969.

568. Borowy, Z. L.: Primary hyperparathyroidism. *Canad J Surg, 12:*104, 1969.

569. Cervela, L. A., Troncoso, Ploa, S., *et al.*: Zollinger-Ellison syndrome. *Rev Clin Esp, 113:*63, 1969.

570. Chkheidze, M. I. A.: (A case of Zollinger-Ellison syndrome.) *Khirurgiia (Moskva), 45:*114, 1969.

571. Creutzfeldt, W.: Zollinger-Ellison syndrome. *Verh Deutsch Ges Inn Med, 75:*242, 1969.

572. Creutzfeldt, W., Creutzfeldt, C., and Perings, E.: Light and electron microscopic findings in three clinical cases of the Zollinger-Ellison syndrome. In Demling, L. and Ottenjann, R. (Eds.): *Non-Insulin Producting Tumors of the Pancreas.* Stuttgart, Georg Thieme Verlag, 86, 1969.

573. Chisholm, D. J., Young, J. D., and Lazarus, L.: The gastrointestinal stimulus to insulin release. *J Clin Invest, 48:*1453, 1969.

574. Debray, C., Hardouin, J. P., and Vasseur, B.: Demonstration of gastro-secretogogue activity of pancreatic origin. Apropos of a case of insulinoma and 3 cases of Zollinger-Ellison syndrome. *Ann Intern Med (Paris), 120:*37, 1969.

575. Desai, H. G., and Antia, F. P.: Spontaneous achlorhydria with atrophic gastritis in the Zollinger-Ellison syndrome. *Gut, 10:*935, 1969.

576. Eckmann, L.: Ulcerative tumors and duodenal ulcer. *Schweiz Med Wochenschr, 99:*852, 1969.

577. Emas, S., Vagne, M., and Grossman, M.: Heidenhain pouch response to antral stimulation before and after antral denervation in dogs. *Fed Proc, 132:*1162, 1969.

578. Emmrich, J., and Frerichs, H.: Clinical and angiographic findings in islet cell adenoma. *Cesk Radiol, 23:*193, 1969.

579. Ferrero, R., and Poletti, G. A.: Zollinger-Ellison syndrome. Case report. *Arch Sci Med (Torino), 123:*1012, 1969.

580. Fongi, E. G., Lagioia, R., Munist, L., *et al.*: Ulcerogenic tumor of the pancreas. Zollinger-Ellison syndrome. *Prensa Med Argent, 56:*375, 1969.

581. Gall, F.: Endocrine pancreatic tumors. Diagnosis and surgical therapy. *Munchen Med Wschr, 111:*682, 1969.

582. Grundner, H. G., Bohm, N., Bohm, N., *et al.*: Multiple endocrine hyperplasias and adenomas associated with Zollinger-Ellison syn-

drome and general thrombosis susceptibility. *Deutsch Med Wochenschr, 94:*375, 1969.
583. Guillard, J., Hivet, M., Lavame, Mme., *et al.:* Limits of the Zollinger-Ellison syndrome. *Arch Fr Mal App Dig, 58:*469, 1969.
584. Isenberg, J. I., Stening, G. F., Ward, S., *et al.:* Relation of gastric secretory response in man to dose of insulin. *Gastroenterology, 57:* 395, 1969.
585. Johnson, L. R., Aures, Dorothea, Hakanson, R.: Effect of gastrin on the in vivo incorporation of 14C-leucine into protein in the digestive tract (34353). *Proc Soc Exp Biol Med, 132:*996, 1969.
586. Johnson, L. R., and Grossman, M.: Potentiation of gastric acid response in the dog. *Gastroenterology, 56:*687, 1969.
587. Kelly, P., and Robert, A.: Inhibition by pregnancy and lactation of steroid-induced ulcers in the rat. *Gastroenterology, 56:*24, 1969.
588. Kluck, J. J., Jr., and Hardy, J. D.: The Zollinger-Ellison syndrome—with report of illustrative case. *J Mississippi Med Ass, 10:*535, 1969.
589. Konturek, S. J., Dubiel, J.: Effect of diversion of bile and pancreatic juice on pentagastrin-produced duodenal ulcers in cats. *Scand J Gastroent, 4:*59, 1969.
590. Lawrence, A. M.: Immunoassays in the diagnoses of endocrine diso-orders. *Surg Clin N Am, 49:*3, 1969.
591. LeBriggs, R., and Powell, J. R.: Chiari-Frommel syndrome as a part of the Zollinger-Ellison multiple endocrine adenomatosis complex. *Calif Med, 111:*92, 1969.
592. Lescut, J., Cerf, M., Bourgeois, J., *et al.:* Diarrhea revealing a Zollinger-Ellison syndrome with gastrojejunitis without ulcer. *Lille Med, 14:* 429, 1969.
593. Manfred, C., *et al.:* Steatorrhea and gastric hypersecretion (experimental study on dogs). *G Ital Chir, 25:*161, 1969.
594. Mason, M. C., and Clark, C. G.: Surgery for duodenal ulcer. *Brit J Surg, 56:*815, 1969.
595. Meeroff, J. C.: Strom-Zollinger-Ellison's syndrome. Ulcerogenic pancreatic syndrome. *Rev Esp Enferm Apar Dig, 28:*675, 1969.
596. Mercadier, M., Bernier, J. J., Melliere, D., *et al.:* Diagnostic problems of the Zollinger-Ellison syndrome without ulcer. Apropos of a further case. *Sem Hop Paris, 45:*3362, 1969.
597. Morgan, E. S.: Surgical treatment of peptic ulcer. *Amer Surg, 35:*805, 1969.
598. Moritz, M., Kahn, P. C., Callow, A. D., *et al.:* Unusual clinical manifestations and angiographic findings in a patient with the Zollinger-Ellison syndrome. *Ann Intern Med, 71:*1133, 1969.
599. Nagele, E.: Radiographic findings in the carcinoid and Zollinger-Ellison syndrome. *Verh Deutsch Ges Inn Med, 75:*675, 1969.
600. Paris, J., Benoit, M., Lagache, G., *et al.:* Zollinger-Ellison syndrome

in diarrheic form and with duodenal adenomatous reaction. *Lille Med, 14:*425, 1969.

601. Penco, T., *et al.:* Functioning and non-functioning tumors of the insular pancreas. Pathology, clinical aspects and therapy. *Osp Ital Chir Suppl, 13:*1, 1969.
602. Phillips, S., and Schmid, W.: Jejunal transport of electrolytes and water in intestinal disease. *Gut, 10:*990, 1969.
603. Pinakapani, S., Pai, K. R., Devi, C. S., *et al.:* Multiple endocrine adenoma peptic ulcer complex. Clinicopathological study of a case. *J Ass Phys India, 17:*105, 1969.
604. Qvist, G., Davis, H., and Fox, J. A.: Conservative surgery for peptic ulcer. *Brit J Clin Pract, 23:*483, 1969.
605. Robnett, A., Durham, M., Harper, H., *et al.:* Second gastric resection for recurrent peptic ulcer. *Am J Surg, 35:*801, 1969.
606. Sircus, W.: Peptide-secreting tumors with special reference to the pancreas. *Gut, 10:*506, 1969.
607. Siurala, M., Rasanen, T., and Varis, K.: The response of human gastric tissue eosinophils to ACTH infusion and to long-term treatment with prednisone. *Scand J Gastroent, 4:*209, 1969.
608. Solcia, E., Vassallo, G., and Capella, C.: Studies on the G cells of the pyloric mucosa, the probable site of gastrin secretion. *Gut, 10:*379, 1969.
609. Stadelmann, O., Elster, K., and Chi, P. H.: Results of endoscopic gastric biopsy. Report on approximately 1500 spot biopsies. *Deutsch Med Wochenschr, 94:*839, 1969.
610. Stening, G., Frank, I., and Jon, I.: Insulin-induced acid secretion after partial vagotomy in dogs and cats. *Am J Physiol, 217:*962, 1969.
611. Strohmeyer, G.: Diagnostic tests for the Zollinger-Ellison syndrome. *German Med Monthly, 14:*93, 1969.
612. Thompson, J. C.: Gastrin and gastric secretion. *Ann Rev Med, 20:*291, 1969.
613. Tsuchiya, M., Ishii, H., Murai, S., *et al.:* Case of insulinoma with multiple stomach ulcer in an aged woman. *Saishin Igaku, 24:*893, 1969.
614. Tuzhilan, S. A., Zhurbin, L. E., and Chepyzhova, V. S.: A case of Zollinger-Ellison syndrome. *Soviet Med, 32:*112, 1969.
615. Vagne, M., and Grossman, M.: Gastric and pancreatic secretion in response to gastric distention in dogs. *Gastroenterology, 57:*300, 1969.
616. Wilken, B. J., Hardy, J. D., Turner, M. D., *et al.:* Bioassay in the diagnosis of the Zollinger-Ellison syndrome. *Ann Surg, 170:*922, 1969.
617. Wohlgemuth, B., *et al.:* Zollinger-Ellison syndrome. *Arch Geschwulstforsch, 33:*132, 1969.
618. Zakelj, V., Matko, I., and Ferluga, D.: The Zollinger-Ellison syndrome

in ectopic ulcerogenic pancreatic neoplasm in the liver. *Med Welt, 30:*1642, 1969.

1970

619. Aliev, S. H. A., Ryskulova, K. R., and Zubekhina, L. M.: Total gastrectomy in Zollinger-Ellison syndrome. *Sov Zdravookhr Kirg, 3:* 56, 1970.
620. Ament, M. E., *et al.:* Zollinger-Ellison syndrome. *J Pediat, 76:*484, 1970.
621. Babb, R. R.: Diagnosis of Zollinger-Ellison syndrome. Ulcerogenic tumor of the pancreas. *Calif Med, 113:*1, 1970.
622. Basso, N., and Passaro, E.: Calcium-stimulated gastric secretion in the Zollinger-Ellison syndrome. *Arch Surg, 101:*399, 1970.
623. Bonfils, S., *et al.:* Recent aspects of Zollinger-Ellison syndrome. *Brux Med, 50:*1087, 1970.
624. Brooks, A., Marvin, J., Leonard, R., *et al.:* Failure of desulfated caerulein to inhibit pentagastrin-stimulated acid secretion. *Am J Physiol, 219:*794, 1970.
625. Brooks, J., and Grossman, M. I.: Effect of combinations of histamine and pentagastrin on gastric secretion in man and dog. *Gastroenterology, 58:*470, 1970.
626. Catt, K. J.: Hormones in general-I. ABC of endocrinology. *Lancet,* 1:7650, 1970.
627. Cavina, X., *et al.:* La prova biologica nella diagnosi della sindrome di Zollinger-Ellison. *Estratto da Chirurgia Gastroenterologica,* Vol. 1, Fasc. I—Gennaio-Marzo.
628. Creutzfeldt, W., Feurle, G., and Ketterer, H.: Effect of gastrointestinal hormones on insulin and glucagon secretion. *New Eng J Med, 282:*1139, 1970.
629. Deucher, F., *et al.:* The Zollinger-Ellison syndrome. *Ther Umsch, 27:* 233, 1970.
630. Dragstedt, L.: Hollander test unnecessary. *JAMA, 212:*320, 1970.
631. Egdahl, R. H.: Surgery of the parathyroid glands. *Surg Gynec Obstet, 130:*901, 1970.
632. Fletcher, J. R.: Medullary (Solid) carcinoma of the thyroid gland. *Arch Surg, 100:*357, 1970.
633. Friesen, S. R., *et al.:* Serum gastrin levels in malignant Zollinger-Ellison syndrome after total gastrectomy and hypophysectomy. *Ann Surg, 172:*504, 1970.
634. Gray, R. K., Rosch, J., and Grollman, J. H., Jr.: Arteriography in the diagnosis of islet-cell tumors. *Radiology, 97:*39, 1970.
635. Greider, M. H., Bencosme, S. A., and Lechago, J.: The human pancreatic islet cells and their tumors. *Lab Invest, 22:*344, 1970.
636. Grossman, M. I.: Hormone-hormone and vagus-hormone interactions on gastric acid secretion. Nobel symposium XVI: Frontiers in gastrointestinal hormone research. Stockholm, July 20–21, 1970.

637. Grossman, M. I.: Proposal: use the term cholecystokinin in place of cholecystokinin-pancreozymin. *Gastroenterology, 58:*128, 1970.

638. Hirata, Y.: Langerhans' cell tumor. *Clin Endocrinol (Tokyo), 18:*1028, 1970.

639. Isaza, J., Sugawara, K., Tiongco, R., *et al.:* Studies of effect of 2-phenyl-2(2-pyridyl)-thioacetami de (antigastrin) on canine gastric acid secretion. *Surgery, 67:*462, 1970.

640. Jesseph, J. E., and Zollinger, R. M.: Surgical treatment of multiglandular syndromes. In Irvin, W. T. (Ed.): Modern trends in surgery-3. London: Butterworth, 150–164, 1970.

641. Jirasek, V.: Relation of Zollinger-Ellison syndrome to multiple endocrinous adenomatosis. Deliberations on the pathogenesis of various forms of peptic ulcer. *Cesk Gastroenterol Vyz, 24:*258, 1970.

642. Johnson, L. R., Stening, G. F., and Grossman, M. I.: Effect of sulfation on the gastrointestinal actions of caerulein. *Gastroenterology, 58:* 208, 1970.

643. Jones, B. S., O'Hagen, J. J., Phear, D. N., *et al.:* A case of the Zollinger-Ellison syndrome associated with hyperplasia of salivary and Brunner's glands. *Gut, 11:*837, 1970.

644. Jones, R. S., and Grossman, M. I.: Choleretic effects of cholecystokinin, gastrin II, and caerulein in the dog. *Am J Physiol, 219:* 1014, 1970.

645. Kocandrle, V., *et al.:* Pulmonary resection for metastasis in non-beta islet cell tumor of pancreas. *Ann Surg, 172:*49, 1970.

646. Korman, M. G., John, D. J., and Hansky, J.: Studies on serum gastrin levels in pernicious anaemia. *Gut, 11:*981, 1970.

647. Kubota, Y.: Cancer of the Langerhans Islands. *Naika, 26:*283, 1970.

648. Levine, R. J., Vaidya, A., Sherman, D. J. C., *et al.:* Effects of brocresine on Zollinger-Ellison syndrome. Report of two cases. *Am J Dig Dis, 15:*477, 1970.

649. Matsuoka, T., Sasano, N., and Miura, K.: Zollinger-Ellison syndrome. *Jap J Cancer Clin, 16:*872, 1970.

650. McGuigan, J. E., and Trudeau, W. L.: Studies with antibodies to gastrin. Radioimmunoassay in human serum and physiological studies. *Gastroenterology, 58:*139, 1970.

651. Meyer, J. H., Way, L. W., and Grossman, M. I.: Pancreatic bicarbonate response to various acids in duodenum of the dog. *Am J Physiol, 219:*964, 1970.

652. Meyer, J. H., Way, L. W., and Grossman, M. I.: Pancreatic response to acidification of varying lengths of proximal intestine in dog. *Am J Physiol, 219:*971, 1970.

653. Neef, J. C., DeKrull, G. H., Vonk, J., *et al.:* Zollinger-Ellison syndrome in a patient with secondary amenorrhea—report of a case with fatal outcome. *Fertil Steril, 21:*43, 1970.

654. Oda, M., and Koshi, J.: Zollinger-Ellison syndrome. *Jap J Clin Med, 28:* 2383, 1970.
655. Okubo, T., Hisama, S., Fujisawa, S., *et al.:* Experience in Zollinger-Ellison syndrome. *Shujutsu, 24:*1325, 1970.
656. Passaro, E., Jr., Basso, N., Sanchez, R. E., *et al.:* Newer studies in the Zollinger-Ellison syndrome. *Am J Surg, 120:*138, 1970.
657. Patterson, M.: The diagnosis of the Zollinger-Ellison syndrome. *Am J Gastroenterol, 54:*470, 1970.
658. Paulino, F.: Zollinger-Ellison syndrome. *Hospital, 77:*747, 1970.
659. Ptak, T., and Kirsner, J. B.: The Zollinger-Ellison syndrome. Polyendocrine adenomatosis and other endocrine associations with peptic ulcer. *Advances Intern Med, 16:*213, 1970.
660. Reeder, D. D., Jackson, B. M., Ban, J., *et al.:* Influence of hypercalcemia on gastric secretion and serum gastrin concentrations in man. *Ann Surg, 172:*540, 1970.
661. Remine, W., Brown, P., Gomes, M., *et al.:* Polypoid hamartomas of Brunner's glands. *Arch Surg, 100:*313, 1970.
662. Sivash, E. S.: Clinical roentgenodiagnosis of Zollinger-Ellison syndrome. *Vestn Rentgenol Radiol, 45:*43, 1970.
663. Small, W., and Jahadi, M. R.: Pyloroplasty and vagotomy for duodenal ulcer. *Amer J Surg, 119:*372, 1970.
664. Sugawara, K., Isaza, J., Curt, J., *et al.:* Distention of the pyloric antrum as a stimulus for gastrin release. *Arch Surg, 100:*201, 1970.
665. Thomson, C. G., Cleator, I. G., and Sircus, W.: Experiences with a rat bioassay in the diagnosis of the Zollinger-Ellison syndrome. *Gut, 11:*409, 1970.
666. Thorbjarnarson, B., and Zahn, F. G.: Total gastrectomy for malignant Zollinger-Ellison syndrome. *New York J Med, 70:*316, 1970.
667. Vachon, A., Tete, R., Spay, G., *et al.:* Anatomo-clinical case of ulcerogenic pancreatic tumor. *Rev Lyon Med, 19:*645, 1970.
668. Wormsley, K. G.: Response to duodenal acidification in man. II. Effects on the gastric secretory response to pentagastrin. *Scand J Gastroent, 5:*207, 1970.
669. Wright, H. K., *et al.:* Impaired intestinal absorption in the Zollinger-Ellison syndrome independent of gastric hypersecretion. *Amer J Surg, 119:*250, 1970.
670. Yalow, R. S., and Berson, S. A.: Size and charge distinctions between endogenous human plasma gastrin in peripheral blood and heptadecapeptide gastrins. *Gastroenterology, 58:*609, 1970.
671. Zhdanov, G. G., and Kotov, I. A.: Zollinger-Ellison syndrome. *Khirurgiia (Mosk),46:*142, 1970.
672. Zollinger, R. M.: Hormone-producing tumors of the pancreas. *Bull Mason Clin, 24:*1, 1970.
673. Zollinger, R. M.: Non-beta islet cell tumors. Current concepts. *J S Carolina Med Ass, 66:*273, 1970.

674. Zollinger, R. M.: The GI effects of pancreatic tumors. *Philadelphia Med, 66:*220, 1970.

1971

675. Acky, R. A., and Knopp, R. H.: Current concepts: evaluation of islet cell function in man. *New Eng J Med, 285:*1130–1131, 1971.
676. Berson, S., and Yalow, Rosalyn: Nature of immunoreactive gastrin extracted from tissues of gastrointestinal tract. *Gastroenterology, 60:*215, 1971.
677. Buchta, R. M., *et al.:* Zollinger-Ellison syndrome in a nine-year-old child: A case report and review of the entity in childhood. *Pediatrics, 47:*594, 1971.
678. Chartaughchawong, S.: An interesting case of Zollinger-Ellison syndrome. *Ariz Med, 28:*292, 1971.
679. Christophersen, L.: The Zollinger-Ellison syndrome. *Ugeskr Laeger, 133:*987, 1971.
680. Croisier, J. C., Lehy, T., and Zeitoun, P.: A2 cell pancreatic microadenomas in a case of multiple endocrine adenomatosis. *Cancer, 28:* 707, 1971.
683. Creutzfeldt, W., *et al.:* Clinical syndromes of hormonally active pancreatic tumors. *Chirurg, 42:*97, 1971.
684. Croisier, J. C., Azerad, E., and Lubetzki, J.: Polyendocrine adenomatosis (Wermer's syndrome). Apropos of a personal case. Review of the literature. *Sem Hop Paris, 47:*494, 1971.
685. Dodds, W. J., Dehn, T. G., Hogan, W. J., *et al.:* Severe peptic esophagitis in a patient with Zollinger-Ellison syndrome. *Am J Roentgenol Radium Ther Nucl Med, 113:*237, 1971.
686. Doolas, A.: Steps in the diagnosis of 3 functioning endocrine tumors. *Surg Clin N Am, 51:*195, 1971.
687. Drage, A. C.: Zollinger-Ellison syndrome. *Nurs Mirror, 132:*38, 1971.
688. Dyck, W. P.: Pancreatic hypersecretion in Zollinger-Ellison syndrome. Case report. *Gastroenterology, 60:*90, 1971.
689. Enderlin, F.: Some aspects of the Zollinger-Ellison syndrome from the surgical viewpoint. *Chirurg, 42:*106, 1971.
690. Espenschade, P. W., Jr., Westminster, M. D.: Letter to Editor. *Amer Med News,* Feb. 22, 1971.
691. Ganguli, P. C., Cullen, D. R., and Irvine, W. J.: Radioimmunoassay of plasmagastrin in pernicious anaemia, hypochlorhydria, and in controls. *Lancet,* 1:155, 1971.
692. Hight, D., James, L. P., and Jahadi, M. R.: Pancreatic islet hyperplasia as a cause of a severe ulcer diathesis. *Arch Surg, 103:*98, 1971.
693. Hivet, M., Moinet, P., Lagadec, B., *et al.:* Zollinger-Ellison syndrome in duodenal aberrant pancreas. Ulcerogenic tumor of the duodenum (Apropos of 5 cases) (Fre). *Am Chir, 25:*883, 1971.
694. Isenberg, J. I., *et al.:* Gastro-esophageal sphincter pressure in pernicious anemia and Zollinger-Ellison syndrome. *Lancet, 1:*972, 1971.

695. Kaplan, E. L., Hill, Barbara J., Locke, Susan, *et al.*: Acid-base balance and parathyroid function—metabolic alkalosis and hyperparathyroidism. *Surgery, 70:*2, 1971.
696. Korman, M. G., Soveny, C., and Hansky, J.: Radioimmunoassay of gastrin. *Scand J Gastroent, 6:*71, 1971.
697. McGuigan, J., and Greider, Marie: Correlative immunochemical and light microscopic studies of the gastrin cell of the antral mucosa. *Gastroenterology, 60:*223, 1971.
698. Murray-Lyon, I. M., Cassar, J., Coulson, R., *et al.*: Further studies on streptozotocin therapy for a multiple-hormone-producing islet cell carcinoma. *Gut, 12:*717, 1971.
699. Oppermann, A., Gradmottet, P., and Carbillet, J. P., *et al.*: Multiple gastric ulcers and pancreatic tumor. *Lyon Med 225:*12, 1971.
700. Rehfeld, J. F., *et al.*: Zollinger-Ellison syndrome. A review. *Ugeskr Laeger, 133:*979, 1971.
701. Shum, H. Y., O'Neill, B. J., and Streeter, A. M.: Vitamin-B12 absorption and the Zollinger-Ellison syndrome. *Lancet, 1:*1303, 1971.
702. Stadil, F., *et al.*: Diagnosis of the Zollinger-Ellison syndrome. Value of serum gastrin determination. *Ugeskr Laeger, 133:*983, 1971.
703. Stadil, F., and Rehfeld, J. F.: Radioimmunoassay of gastrin in human serum. *Scand J Gastroenterol,* 6 suppl, 9:61-5, 1971.
704. Stadil, F., Rehfeld, J. F., and Thaysen, E. H.: Gastric juice as gastrin-releasing factor in the Zollinger-Ellison syndrome. *Lancet, 2:*102, 1971.
705. Trudeau, W. L., *et al.*: Relations between serum gastrin levels and rates of gastric hydrochloric acid secretion. *New Eng J Med, 284:* 408, 1971.
706. Trudeau, W., McGuigan, J.: Serum gastrin levels and rates of gastric hydrochloric acid secretion. *New Eng J Med, 284:*408, 1971.
707. Vaidya, A. B., *et al.*: Effects of anticholinergic drugs on Zollinger-Ellison syndrome. *Am J Dig Dis, 16:*657, 1971.
708. Vogel, T. T.: Notes on Streptozotocin in metastatic insulinoma. *J Surg Oncol, 3:*481, 1971.
709. Wilson, S. D., Schulte, W. J., and Meade, R. C.: Longevity studies following total gastrectomy in children with the Zollinger-Ellison syndrome. *Arch Surg, 103:*108, 1971.
710. Yalow, Rosalyn, and Berson, S.: Further studies on the nature of immunoreactive gastrin in human plasma. *Gastroenterology, 60:* 203, 1971.
711. Weichert, R. F., Roth, L. W., Kremetz, E. T., *et al.*: Carcinoid islet cell tumors of the duodenum. Report of 21 cases. *Amer J Surg, 121:* 196, 1971.
712. Zollinger, R. M.: Gastrin, Clinical Evaluation of Hormonal Excess. In Berson, S. A. (Ed.): *Methods of Investigative and Diagnostic Endocrinology.* Amsterdam: North Holland, in press.

713. Zollinger, R. M., Vogel, T. T., and Sherman, N. J.: Post-resectional gastrojejunocolic fistula with perforation and Zollinger-Ellison tumor. In Hardy, J. D. (Ed.): Critical surgical illness. Philadelphia: Saunders, 1971.
714. Zollinger, R. M.: 13 unpublished cases.

ADDITIONAL READINGS

1902

715. Bayliss, W., and Starling, E. H.: The mechanism of pancreatic secretion. *J Physiol, 28:*3251, 1902.

1903

716. Erdheim, J.: Fur normalen und pathologischen histologic der glandula thyroidea, parathyreoidea und hypophysis. *Beitr Path Anat, 33:* 158, 1903.

1905

717. Starling, E. H.: The chemical control of the functions of the body. *Lancet, 2:*339, 1905.
718. Starling, E. H.: The chemical reflexes of the alimentary tract. *Lantern, 2:*501, 1905.

1906

719. Edkins, J. S.: The chemical mechanism of gastric secretion. *J Physiol, (London), 34:*133, 1906.

1911

720. Exalto, J.: Ulcus jejuni nach Gastroenterostomie, Mitt a.d. Granzgeb. d. *Med Chir, 23:*13, 1911.

1923

721. Mann, F. C., and Williamson, C. S.: The experimental production of peptic ulcer. *Ann Surg, 77:*409, 1923.

1930

722. Dragstedt, L. R., Montgomery, M. L., and Ellis, J. C.: A new type of pancreatic fistula. *Proc Soc Exp Biol Med, 28:*109, 1930.

1931

723. Connell, F. G.: Fundusectomy experimental. *Surg Gynec Obstet, 53:* 750, 1931.
724. Elman, R., and Hartman, A. F.: Spontaneous peptic ulcers of duodenum after continued loss of pancreatic juice. *Arch Surg, 23:* 1030, 1931.

1935

725. Seely, H., and Zollinger, R. M.: Fundusectomy in the treatment of peptic ulcer. *Surg Gynec Obstet, 61:*155, 1935.

1938

726. Sandweiss, D. N., Sahzstein, H. C., and Farbmann, A.: The prevention

of healing of experimental peptic ulcer in Mann-Williamson Dogs with the anterior pituitary-like hormone (Antuitrin-S). *Am J Dig Dis, 5:*24, 1938.

727. Whipple, A. O.: The surgical therapy of hyperinsulinism. *J Int Chir, 3:* 237, 1938.

1942

728. Dragstedt, L. R.: Pathogenesis of gastroduodenal ulcer. *Arch Surg, 44:* 438, 1942.
729. Hay, L. J., Varco, R. L., Code, C. F., and Wangensteen, O. H.: Experimental production of gastric and duodenal ulcers in laboratory animals by intramuscular injection of histamine in beeswax. *Surg Gynec Obstet, 75:*170, 1942.

1948

730. Poth, E. J., Manhoff, L. J., and DeLoach, A. W.: The relation of pancreatic secretion to peptic ulcer formation. Effect of pancreatectomy, ligation of pancreatic ducts and diabetes on the production of histamine-induced ulcers in the dog. *Surgery, 24:*62, 1948.

1950

731. Brown, C. H., Neville, W. E., and Hazard, J. B.: Islet-cell adenoma, without hypoglycemia, causing duodenal obstruction. *Surgery, 27:* 616, 1950.

1951

732. Janowitz, H. D., and Crohn, B. B.: Hyperinsulinism and duodenal ulcer—a rare clinical combination. *Gastroenterology, 17:*578, 1951.

1952

733. Forty, F., and Barrett, G. M.: Peptic ulceration of the third part of the duodenum associated with islet-cell tumours of the pancreas. *Brit J Surg, 40:*60, 1952–53.
734. Strom, R.: A case of peptic ulcer and insulinoma. *Acta Chir Scand, 104:*252, 1952.

1953

735. Underdahl, L. O., Woolner, L. B., and Black, B. M.: Multiple endocrine adenomas: Report of 8 cases in which the parathyroids, pituitary and pancreatic islets were involved. *J Clin Endocr, 13:*20, 1953.

1954

736. Wermer, P.: Genetic aspects of adenomatosis of endocrine glands. *Am J Med, 16:*363, 1954.

Section II

THE DIARRHEOGENIC SYNDROME

INTRODUCTION

NON-BETA ISLET CELL TUMORS of the pancreas have been associated with diarrhea for at least a quarter of a century. A diarrheogenic hormone of islet cell origin was first postulated in 1961[19] to explain certain cases of intractable diarrhea in which gastric hypersecretion was not a factor. Seven years later, it was suggested that the diarrheogenic hormone is secretin, or a secretin-like substance.[46] This observation was based on extensive clinical and laboratory studies of two patients with the clinical triad of watery diarrhea, hypokalemia, and achlorhydria—known by some as pancreatic cholera and by others as the WDHA syndrome.[28,34] A suitable name to describe this syndrome has not yet been generally accepted; and recent studies by Sircus and by Grossman have raised the question of *multiple* humoral factors (gastrin-glucagon-secretin) being responsible for the individual aspects of this polymorphous disease.[56,58,59] The historical development of the "diarrheogenic syndrome" concept will be presented, with emphasis on the humoral pathogenesis, mechanism of the diarrhea, and deranged calcium homeostasis. For the purposes of this discussion, "diarrheogenic syndrome," "WDHA syndrome," and "pancreatic cholera" will be considered synonymous.

DIARRHEA AND ISLET CELL TUMORS

Gordon and Olivetti, in 1947, first reported the association of pancreatic adenoma and intractable diarrhea. Their patient had diarrhea, a perforated esophageal ulcer, and three chronic duodenal ulcers associated with multiple pancreatic and adrenocortical adenomas.[2] In 1950, Brown, Neville, and Hazard described a 74-year-old woman who had diarrhea and an islet cell tumor but neither peptic ulcer nor hypoglycemia.[3] She became asymptomatic after removal of a 78 gm tumor. Intractable diarrhea developed one year before peptic ulceration in a case reported by Forty and Barrett.[6] This patient was subsequently found to have multiple pancreatic adenomas. Likewise, Moldawer, Nardi, and Raker, in 1954, reported a case of diarrhea and renal tubular changes suggestive of hypokalemia associated with a large islet cell tumor.[7]

Although one of the two original ulcerogenic tumor patients had diarrhea for eight years before the diagnosis of peptic ulcer, it was not emphasized, since the authors wished to keep their clinical findings in a triad.[8] The association was first emphasized as part of the new syndrome two years later when Priest and Alexander (Fig. 56) reported the case of a 59-year-old woman who presented such serious gastrointestinal loss of potassium that she finally died of it, despite massive oral and parenteral replacement therapy.[11] Verner and Morrison (Fig. 57), in 1958, described two similar male patients, one 67 and the other 19 years

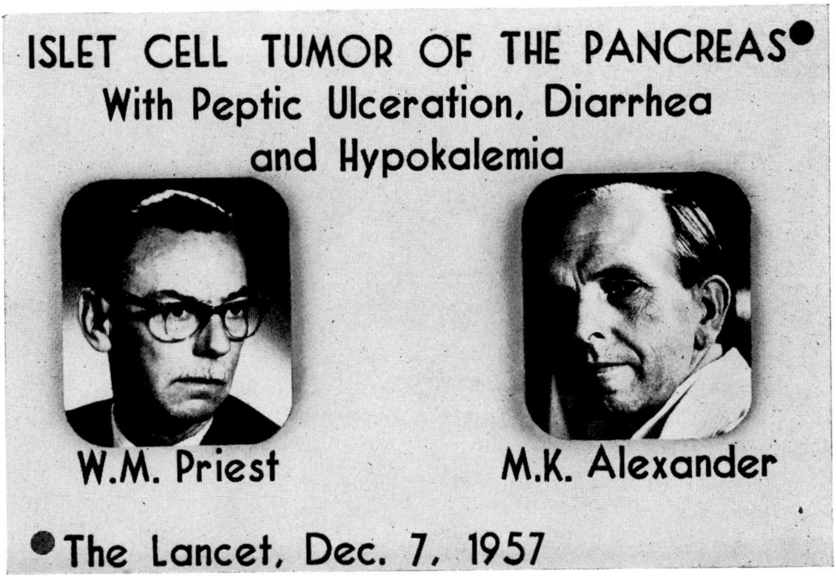

Figure 56. Within two years of the report of the islet cell ulcerogenic syndrome, attention was called to a variation characterized by diarrhea and hypokalemia.

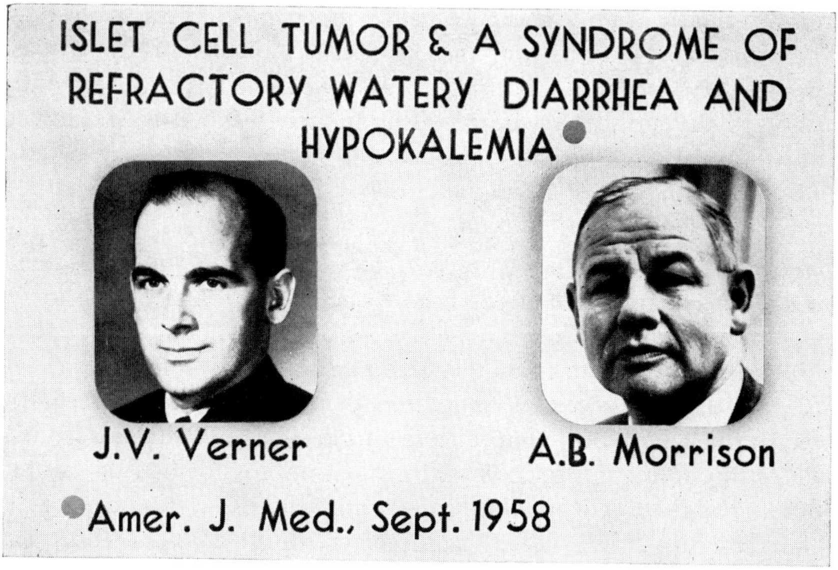

Figure 57. A separate syndrome was developed, characterized by watery diarrhea and hypokalemia without peptic ulceration.

of age, with a syndrome of diarrhea, hypokalemia, and death from renal failure in association with islet cell tumors.[12] These authors also cited seven additional cases from the literature. In the discussion of this important early paper, they made the astute observation that

> It is difficult to say whether peptic ulceration and diarrhea in relation to islet cell adenomas are merely separate expressions of a common determining secretion of the tumor or are more causally related. An attractive but as yet unsubstantiated possibility is that two different tumors of the islets may exist, one composed of alpha cells and the other of delta cells, each associated with a different clinical course; in the one peptic ulcers predominating, in the other diarrhea more in evidence.

With respect to the mechanism of the diarrhea, Verner and Morrison postulated that "The watery nature of the diarrhea is perhaps more compatible with increased production than malabsorption of gastrointestinal juices. . . . It is possible that the tumor may put out some substance causing stimulation of gastrointestinal secretion."

ZOLLINGER-ELLISON AND "NON-SPECIFIC" DIARRHEA RECOGNIZED

From the stimulation of Verner and Morrison's paper, Bruce Charles and his colleagues, in 1960, reported the case of a 34-year-old unmarried woman, which they recognized in retrospect.[14] No measurement of the gastric acid was made, and while the patient did have an esophageal ulcer, they attributed this to extreme vomiting. More importantly, they theorized that "in patients where diarrhea is the chief symptom there may exist an abnormal secretion of some substance from the islet tumor responsible for excess production of succus entericus and hyperperistalsis." Since their patient's tumor was reported to contain islets of the alpha cell type: "It would seem possible, therefore, that one must consider that excess glucagon production may be responsible for the gastrointestinal symptoms present in our patient." That same year, Chears *et al.* of the Baylor University Hospital in Dallas described a case which they felt was the first reported instance in which the diagnosis was made preoperatively and verified at the time of celiotomy.[15] Total removal of a 5 × 7 cm firm, lobulated tumor from the midportion of the body of the pancreas resulted in relief of all symptoms. These authors concluded:

> It seems clear that the absorptive function of the ileum and cecum was insufficient in this patient, leading to the loss of large quantities of fluid. It is a matter of speculation whether this failure of fluid absorption was secondary to an excessive influx by pancreatic or gastrointestinal secretion, exceeding the absorptive capacity of the ileum and cecum, or to inhibition of absorption, perhaps by a humoral substance elaborated by the tumor.

The importance of the acid factor, in these cases the *absence* of gastric hypersecretion, was unfortunately not recognized by these early authors. Thus it was assumed that they were dealing with perhaps a variant of the Zollinger-Ellison syndrome. Gregory and Tracy's monumental finding in 1960[16] that gastrin is the active principal in ulcerogenic tumors was soon extended to provide a sound explanation for the diarrhea on the basis of the marked gastric hypersecretion with neutralization of the pancreatic enzymes and irritation of the mucosa, as well as by direct stimulation of the intestinal tract.[46] As more cases were reported, however, definite irregularities became apparent; and gradually it was appreciated that certain patients with non-beta islet cell tumors did not have gastric hypersecretion and a fulminating ulcer diathesis.

This impression was substantiated by Murray *et al.* in 1961.[18] They documented gastric achlorhydria in a 49-year-old baker with a 16-year history of diarrhea and flushing who was found to have a 5 × 6.5 cm non-beta islet cell adenoma in the tail of the pancreas. The diarrhea stopped abruptly after removal of the adenoma. Clearly, the diarrhea and flushing in this patient was not secondary to gastric hypersecretion, the mechanism which had been suggested as the etiologic factor in the diarrhea of the ulcerogenic syndrome. The authors noted: "Overproduction of succus entericus seems the best explanation of the large volume of diarrhea. . . . A pancreatic hormone causing gastric hypersecretion or diarrhea has as yet not been conclusively demonstrated. . . . This combination of flushing and diarrhea suggested hyperserotenemia to many observers, but laboratory findings did not support this impression."

R. A. Parkins of the Charing Cross Hospital in London described that same year a case in which peptic ulceration was never a feature, and "Hydrochloric acid secretion and the histamine response were poor."[17]

Six years then elapsed before achlorhydria was firmly established as one of the hallmarks of a diarrheal disease of islet cell origin that clearly was not a variant of the Zollinger-Ellison syndrome. In the meantime, however, several important papers were written about the character, etiology, and mechanism of the diarrheogenic syndrome as it is known today.

Telling and Smiddy,[19] in 1961, suggested "either that peptic ulceration is not necessarily part of the Zollinger-Ellison syndrome, which in any case must be enlarged to include diarrhea and steatorrhea, or that *the association of intractable diarrhea, hypokalemia, hyponatremia and islet cell tumors of the pancreas* (excluding those arising in the insulin-secreting beta cells) *constitutes a syndrome entirely distinct from that described by Zollinger and Ellison.*" They also said, "There may be two different types of non–insulin-secreting islet cell tumors of the pancreas: the one may cause gastric over-secretion and peptic ulceration; the other intestinal oversecretion, diarrhea and hypokalemia. How these different reactions are mediated unfortunately remains quite obscure. It is tempting to postulate a hormonal mechanism."

"DIARRHEOGENIC HORMONE" SUGGESTED

In a particularly well documented study, Espiner and Beaven described a case of watery diarrhea and hypokalemia associated with malignant recurrence of a non-beta islet cell tumor.[20] Their patient, a 48-year-old lady, had *complete* achlorhydria, a feature not previously documented as occurring with islet cell tumors. There was striking relief of symptoms with the initial tumor resection, but only temporary improvement in the diarrhea followed similar surgery for a "malignant" adenoma four years later. Tumor extract was tested in an isolated guinea pig ileum preparation, but there was no evidence to support the presence of a substance promoting bowel motility. Likewise, thorough investigation of the patient's small bowel absorptive capacity failed to reveal any impairment. This, together with the normal appearance of small bowel mucosa in biopsy and autopsy material, were felt to mitigate against an absorptive defect for water and electrolytes as the cause of the diarrhea.

The authors measured the output of labeled potassium in the stool and urine of their patient with oral as well as intravenous administration of ^{42}K. The results were compared to those in a normal patient and in a patient with ulcerative colitis and diarrhea. The islet cell tumor patient had a much greater fecal potassium excretion which could not be attributed to an increase in the number or volume of the stools. Furthermore, the recovery of ^{42}K was the same in both the urine and the stool, regardless of the route of administration, indicating that the electrolyte had been completely absorbed. They concluded, "It would not be unreasonable to suggest that a humoral agent of islet origin promotes the secretion of succus entericus," which is also responsible for hypokalemia. The possible role of glucagon was considered, since their patient had reduced glucose tolerance and since her blood glucose levels rose rapidly during surgery when the tumor was being manipulated. Slight hyperglycemic activity was suggested by tumor bioassay in Wistar rats, but there was insufficient extract to replicate the findings.

The association between achlorhydria and biopsy evidence of a normal gastric mucosa first was documented in 1964 by Hindle, McBrien, and Creamer.[26] They concluded that the achlorhydria was due to inhibition of gastric secretion; but the cause of the inhibition was to remain uncertain for several more years.

Yet another aspect of this polymorphous disease was emphasized in 1964 by Brown and Crile. Their patient, a 34-year-old farmer, had a syndrome of profuse diarrhea, hypokalemia, and hypercalcemia associated with parathyroid and pancreatic adenomas.[24] He did not have gastric hypersecretion or peptic ulceration—"differentiating this condition from the Zollinger-Ellison syndrome." More importantly, the authors noted that only temporary remissions in the hypercalcemia were obtained after two operations on the parathyroid glands, while *complete* remission followed subtotal pancreatectomy which removed a 280 gm, 9.5 cm adenoma from the tail of the pancreas. A portion of the tumor was sent to the National Institutes of Health for assay of a possible diarrheogenic substance. No such property could be detected. The authors theorized that

> A simple explanation in our own case would be that the hypercalcemia produced the diarrhea, since each of the three times the hypercalcemia was corrected, the diarrhea stopped. The fact that hypercalcemia recurred with excision of a parathyroid adenoma and also after excision of hyperplasia of the parathyroids, and did not recur with removal of the pancreatic tumor suggests that pancreatic tumors, in addition to parathyroid adenomas, may produce hypercalcemia. These relationships are obscure.

Two years later, Matsumoto (Fig. 58) and colleagues studied such a patient operated upon by Longmire and analyzed 15 additional cases from the English literature. The term, "pancreatic cholera," coined by Mellinkoff, was introduced to characterize this small group of patients[34]: "The term pancreatic "cholera" seems appropriate in its emphasis on this violent and devastating phase of the disease, which if left untreated at this point inevitably results in progressive dehydration, hypokalemia and death."

The 85 gm, well-encapsulated tumor removed from their patient, a 49-year-old female school teacher, did not contain gastrin when assayed by Grossman. Furthermore, an extract of the tumor had no effect on water or glucose transport in a canine small bowel mucosal preparation, nor was there any effect on short circuit current when lyophilized tissue was added to the inside bathing solution of a frog skin preparation. They concluded:

> The circumstantial evidence available strongly suggests that there is a hormone-like substance produced by the islet cell tumor which causes diarrhea. . . . The postulated hormone that produces the syndrome is not gastrin. . . . The mechanism of production of diarrhea remains obscure [although] an excessive secretion of succus entericus would seem the most appealing theory.

Marks (Fig. 58), Bank, and Louw, in 1967, suggested that this disease entity be characterized as an eponym—WDHA syndrome—consisting of its hallmark symptoms: *w*atery *d*iarrhea, *h*ypokalemia, *a*chlorhydria.[40] On the basis of their personal experience with one patient and a review of 15 additional case reports, these

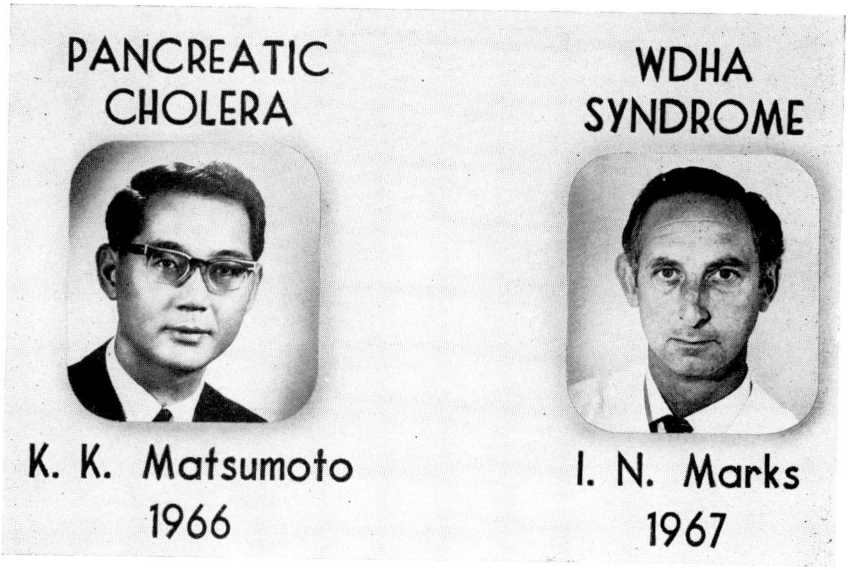

Figure 58. The islet cell tumor associated with watery diarrhea, hypokalemia, and achlorhydria has been designated as pancreatic cholera or the WDHA syndrome in addition to the diarrheogenic syndrome.

authors set forth rather precise criteria for the inclusion of patients in the WDHA category. It was their feeling that the WDHA syndrome could not be diagnosed without documented achlorhydria, marked hyposecretion, or a negative gastrin assay of the tumor extract. Furthermore, reports in which electrolyte levels had not been documented were said to be "presumptive" cases only. On the other hand, they had less to say about the tumor itself: "The pathological features [of this syndrome] are virtually identical with those found in patients with the Zollinger-Ellison syndrome. There are no obvious differences in the gross and histological appearances of the primary or secondary tumors, and in both conditions liver metastases can be shelled quite easily from adjacent liver tissue."

With regard to the etiology and mechanism of the diarrhea,

> Acid hypersecretion does not apply and this, together with the absence of objective evidence of organic disease of the small bowel, makes it difficult to escape the conclusion that the diarrhea is due to an isolated defect of water and electrolyte transport in the bowel, caused by an as yet unidentified islet cell hormone. The watery diarrhea in such patients is unassociated with the loss of gastric electrolytes and characteristically results in hypokalemic acidosis.

Finally, in a series of several companion studies utilizing islet cell carcinoma removed from a 31-year-old pharmaceutical representative, Gardner, Cerda, Peskin, Brooks, and their colleagues were able to extend greatly our understanding of the mechanism of diarrhea in this syndrome.[37,38,53] Their patient had 15 to 40 bowel movements per day with stool volumes as high as 8 liters in 24 hours and hypokalemia but no gastric hypersecretion or peptic ulceration. Balance studies demonstrated excessive fecal losses of fluid and electrolytes. Transit time was normal. Continuous aspiration from the patient's distal ileum demonstrated a pronounced increase in the volume of fluid passing from the small intestine into the colon. *In vitro* studies using a distilled-water extract of an hepatic metastasis demonstrated inhibition of the net mucosal-to-serosal transfer of fluid, sodium, and chloride in an everted hamster gut sac. Intestinal motility was not altered.

Further studies on the effects of gastrin, secretin, and cholecystokinin on *in vitro* fluid and electrolyte transfer were carried out utilizing the small intestine of the hamster as an experimental preparation. It was concluded that:

> The production of a secretin- or cholecystokinlike substance by the tumors of these patients might theoretically result in diarrhea by increasing pancreatic or biliary secretion while decreasing the absorptive capacity of the small intestine for fluid and electrolytes. Production of a secretin-like substance by the tumor is an especially attractive hypothesis for those patients with watery diarrhea and achlorhydria, since it has been demonstrated that secretin can inhibit gastric acid secretion in dogs. . . . Presently, however, there is no evidence for the excessive production of a secretin-, cholecystokinin-, or gastrin-like substance in patients with non-beta islet cell tumors with watery diarrhea without gastric hypersecretion or peptic ulceration Fig. 59.

IDENTIFICATION OF THE DIARRHEOGENIC HORMONE

Marshalling the evidence of these and other experiences, including two personal cases, Zollinger, Tompkins, Amerson, Endahl, Kraft, and Moore (on April 18, 1968, before the American Surgical Association) implicated *secretin* as the diarrheogenic

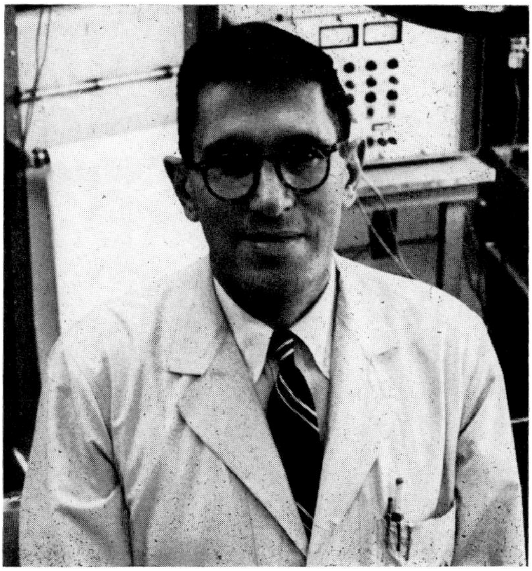

Figure 59. The studies of Dr. Gerald W. Peskin and his associates suggested secretin as the possible hormone produced by the diarrheogenic tumor.

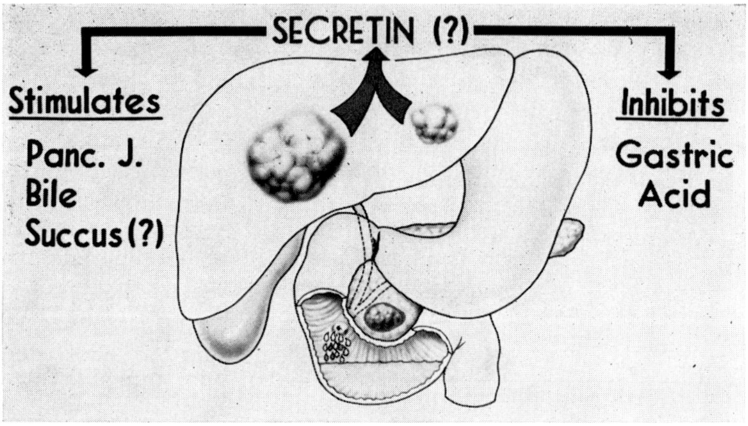

Figure 60. Schematic illustration of the physiological effects produced by the diarrheogenic islet cell tumor and metastasis.

hormone associated with non-beta islet cell tumors of the pancreas (Fig. 60).[46] The reasoning behind this suggestion, as given in the paper, is repeated here *in toto* (Fig. 61).

> Both patients presented with watery diarrhea, hypokalemia and achlorhydria. Gastrin activity was not present in either non-beta islet cell tumor. The first significant clue to secretory overactivity of the

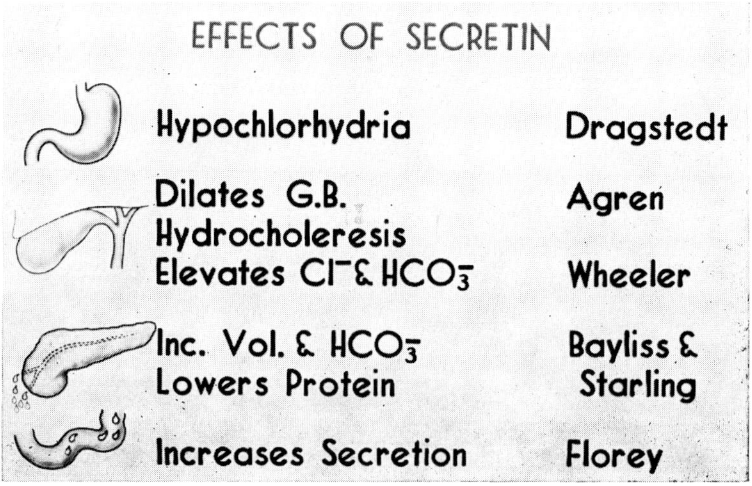

Figure 61. The chemical and laboratory findings in several studied patients are consistent with the effect of secretin as reported by our physiologist.

pancreas and biliary tract in these patients was the observation in Case 1 that the duodenum refilled with secretions during the operative procedure and that the gallbladder was obviously enlarged. Bile was aspirated from the gallbladder for complete chemical analysis in the Biliary Research Laboratory of the Department of Surgery. The unexpected finding of high chloride and bicarbonate levels (Table 1) in the otherwise very dilute bile led to the suspicion that an unusual choleretic agent was being liberated by the islet cell tumor (Figs. 62, 63).

A review of choleretic hormones investigated in the past disclosed that significantly elevated levels of both chloride and bicarbonate in bile had been described only after secretin infusions in animals.[29] Other choleretic hormones such as pancreozymin-cholecystokinin have been shown not to significantly elevate bicarbonate or chloride levels in bile, while it has recently been demonstrated that gastrin significantly raises the bicarbonate concentration but has no effect on the chloride level. Histamine, which has a significant choleretic action, decreases bicarbonate levels while raising the chloride concentrations in bile.[35]

The dilated gallbladder found in Case 1 was quite consistent with observations previously described after secretin administration. This phenomenon is the basis for the secretin test of biliary function in humans.[1] The suggestive chemical findings in the bile of Case 1 prompted the subsequent aspiration of bile for complete analysis

TABLE I
GALLBLADDER BILE ANALYSES

Determinations	*Case 1*	*Case 2*	*Control* *
Sodium (mEq/1)	156	145	187.4 ± 38.7
Potassium (MEq/1)	2.4	2.6	11.5 ± 4.5
Chloride (mEq/1)	111	90	
Bicarbonate (mEq/1)	26.2	48.1	41.6 ± 21.9
Bilirubin, total/direct (mg/100 ml)	52.5/50	9.2/7.4 77.4	8.8 ± 7.9
Bile acids (mEq/1)	**21.2**	9.5	300/-
pH	7.65	7.73	143/ ± 55.9
Osmolality (mOsm/1)	281	276	6.5-9.0
Specific viscosity (Centipoise)	1.029	1,096	300
	(29° C)	(25°)	H20 = 1.000
Specific gravity	1.016	1.010	1.033
Water conc. (gm/100 ml)	97.5	97.5	82
Total solids (gm/100 ml)	3.8	3.8	16.6

* Mean of 10 normal patients.

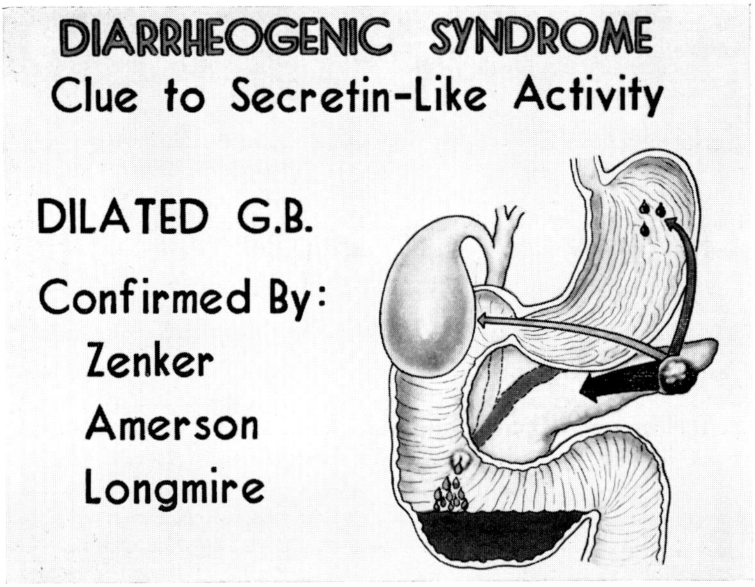

Figure 62. A dilated gallbladder is present in the presence of a diarrheogenic islet cell tumor.

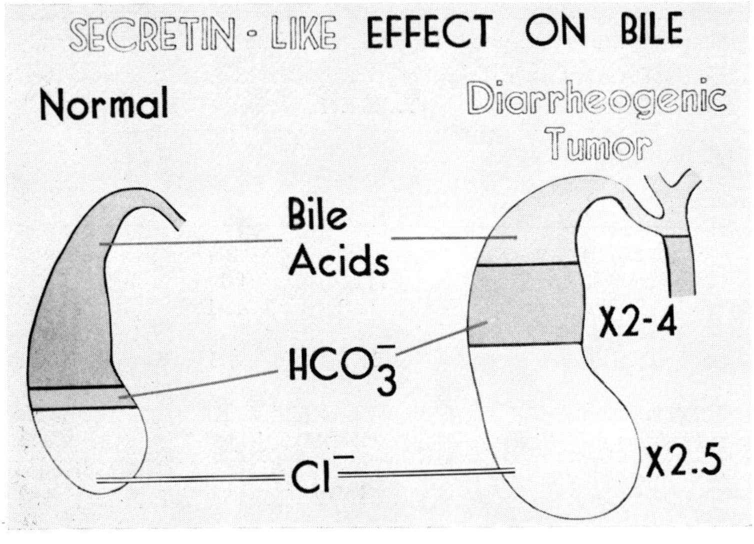

Figure 63. The bile from two cases has shown an increase in chloride and bicarbonate consistent with the effect of secretin.

from the obviously distended gallbladder in Case 2. The strikingly similar chemical results in the bile of the latter case were indeed encouraging (Table I).

The third exciting similarity in both patients was basal achlorhydria, not refractory histamine. The ability to override the achlorhydria in both patients by histamine stimulation suggested that an inhibitory substance might be elaborated by the tumors in these patients. Although postoperative gastric analyses were not performed in Case 2 because of the presence of large amounts of metastatic tumor and because of her early demise, it was possible to carry out several postoperative gastric acid determinations in Case 1. The suprising and prompt return of normal acid values in this patient within 5 days after operation strongly implied that an inhibitory factor had been removed with the excision of the pancreatic tumors. Gastric analysis performed 8½ months after operation continued to show normal amounts of free acid (Table I).

Dragstedt *et al*[10] have demonstrated that secretin inhibits basal gastric acid output as well as acid stimulation by feeding. Similar findings have led Grossman to speculate that secretin might be of eventual value in the treatment of duodenal ulcer. Secretin is not usually able to completely inhibit insulin or histamine-stimulated secretion. However, in 12 proven cases of non-beta islet cell tumors with watery diarrhea, hypokalemia, and achlorhydria collected to date, five of the six patients with malignant islet cell tumors had histamine-fast achlorhydria. This suggests that such malignant tumors may be capable of more marked production of the responsible hormone.

To confirm the presence of secretin, the pancreatic tumor from the senior author's patient (Case 1) (Fig. 64) and the liver metastases removed from Dr. Amerson's patient (Case 2) were prepared for bioassay. The method of extraction, modified for small quantities, was provided by Dr. T. M. Lin (Fig. 65), of Eli Lilly Laboratories in Indianapolis, Indiana.[21] Because of technical objections arising from the use of a chronically prepared, conscious dog, it was decided to employ a modification of the bioassay model suggested by Lin (Fig. 66). The experiments were carried out in a total of 14 mongrel dogs.

Two extracts were prepared from the firm pancreatic tumor of Case 1 and injected three times into two dogs. In the first dog,

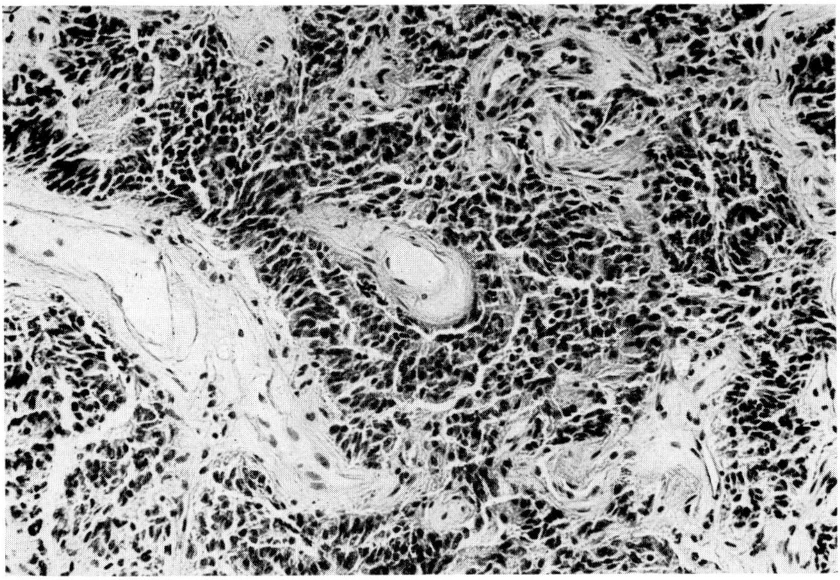

Figure 64. Microscopic examination of the surgically removed pancreas showed the large tumor to be composed of papillary and solid groups of tall columnar cells. The tumor was poorly encapsulated and the cells showed trabecular or rosette-like arrangements.

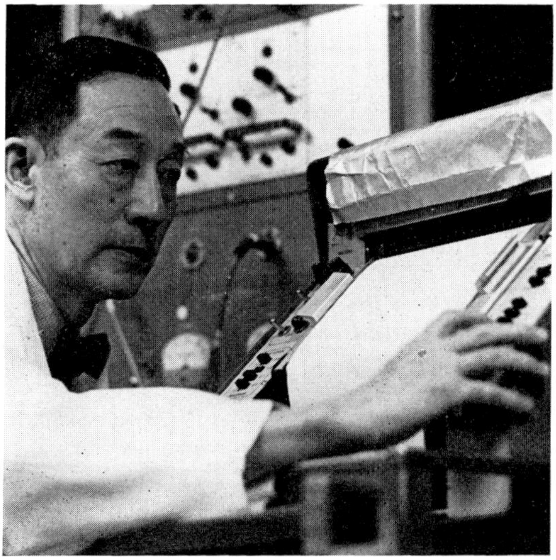

Figure 65. Dr. T. M. Lin has verified the presence of secretin in the bioassay of several diarrheogenic islet cell tumors of the pancreas.

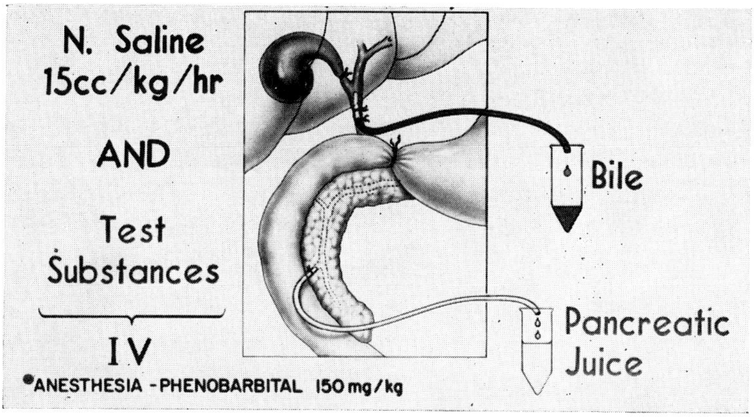

Figure 66. The experimental model, modified from T. M. Lin, for the bioassay of secretin and other test substances in anesthetized dogs.

an extract of 1.6 grams was injected in two equal doses of 800 mg each, with no response. One gram of extract from the same tumor was injected as a single dose in the second dog. Again there was no pancreatic response.

Extracts prepared from the cellular hepatic metastases were

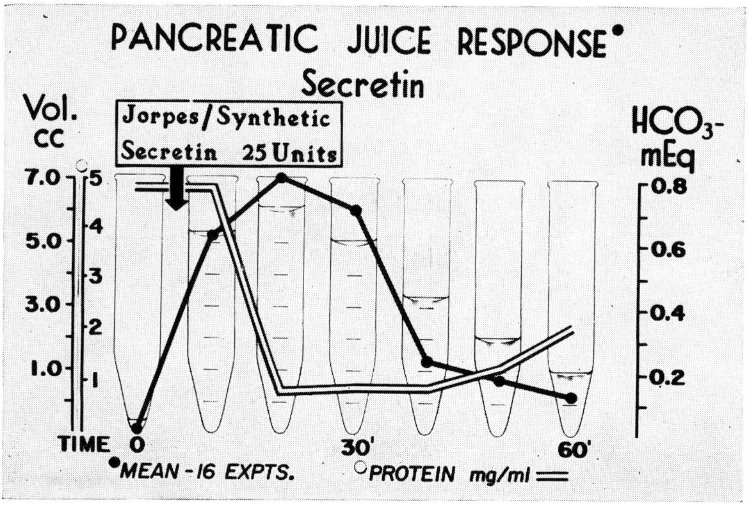

Figure 67. The typical pancreatic juice response to the intravenous injection of Jorpes secretin in the Lin preparation.

tested in these animals. The largest amount of tissue, 178 grams, yielded 7.1 grams of extract. Of this, 500 mg and 450 mg were injected into two dogs and produced a prompt rise in the output of pancreatic juice and bile strikingly similar to that produced by Jorpes secretion (Figs. 67, 68). A third extract, weighing 800 mg, was injected into a third dog and again produced a secretin-like pancreatic response.

In addition to the volume response, there was also a rise in pancreatic juice bicarbonate concentration and output, with a concomitant fall in the concentration and output of chloride. A drop in the enzyme concentration of the pancreatic juice was reflected in the decreased pancreatic juice amylase and total protein concentrations.

Of the control substances tested in the same bioassay preparation (pancreozymin, glucagon, gastrin pentapeptide, histamine, serotonin and prostaglandins) only Jorpes and synthetic secretin evoked a similar pancreatic response (Fig. 69).

The authors theorized that since the pancreatic islet arise embryologically from the dorsal bud of the pancreas, which has a common cell of origin with the antrum and duodenum, "This

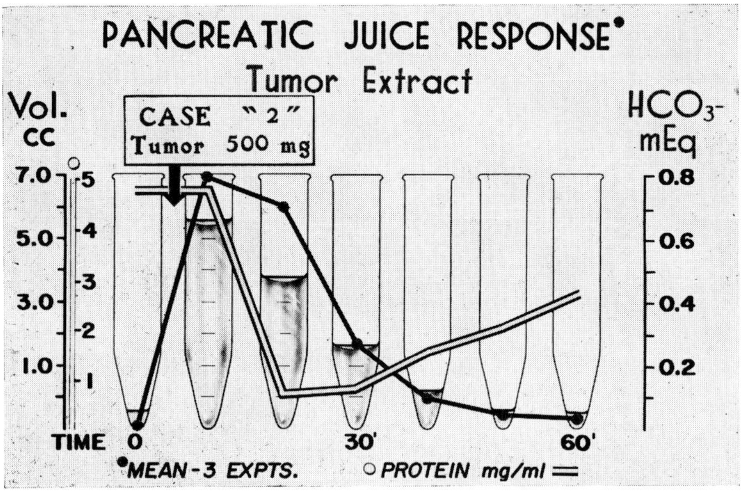

Figure 68. The classical secretin response in the Lin preparation to the injection of an extract of a tumor metastases to the liver.

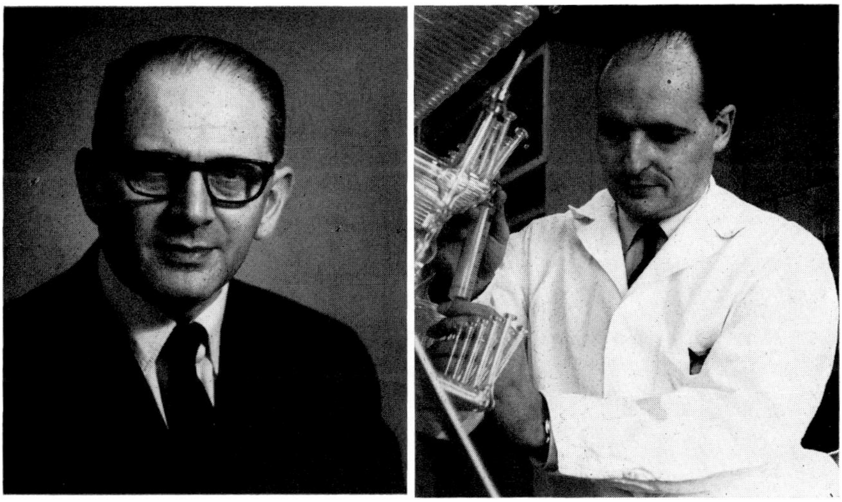

Figure 69. Drs. M. Bodansky and M. A. Ondetti, who synthesized secretin.

provides an anatomical rationale for the production of the antral hormone gastrin, as well as the duodenal hormone secretin, by tumors of these islet cells." Furthermore, recalling the patient of Brown and Crile as well as the later experience of Kofstad *et al.*[39] it was noted that:

> The intriguing observation, in Case 1 of hypercalcemia occurring simultaneously with diarrhea and unrelieved by nearly total parathyroidectomy and the finding at autopsy in Case 2 of uniform parathyroid hyperplasia, raises the possibility of still another hormone being produced by these tumors. In a review of the proven cases . . . over half have shown hypercalcemia which was not necessarily related to the onset of diarrhea.

Tompkins, Kraft, and Zollinger later reported that the effects of these same active extracts upon the flow as well as the bicarbonate and chloride secretion of the hepatic bile in test animals were qualitatively similar to those of Jorpes and synthetic secretin.[50] Thin-layer chromatography of both patients' bile samples was carried out, since it had been reported that cleavage of conjugated bile acids to free bile acids may cause diarrhea. Tompkins reported that "This qualitative test confirmed the normal distribution of bile acids in these patients, i.e. chiefly glycine conjugates with small amounts of taurine conjugates and no detectable free bile acids. Hence, it did not seem likely that the production of free or unusual bile acids by the liver was responsible for the diarrhea in these patients."

Diarrhea could not previously be produced in conscious dogs despite constant intravenous infusion of as much as 35 units of Jorpes secretin per kilogram per hour for as long as 53 hours. Explosive diarrhea did occur, however, in two conscious animals receiving continuous intravenous secretin, after rapid intravenous administration of the active tumor extract. Tompkins was able to obtain additional information on this physiologic effect of secretin by administering intravenously 1 unit/kg of Jorpes secretin to a 75 kg fasting female. This subject had had an indwelling T-tube placed during choledochotomy several days previously. Total bile collection was possible during the base-line and secretin-stimulated periods by inflating the balloon on the distal end of the Baldwin-type T-tube. The characteristic increases in bile volume, bicarbonate, and chloride secretion were observed. More important, however, this lady had the onset of explosive watery diarrhea approximately four hours later, a side effect observed by Wormsley in his clinical study on the effects of secretin in man.[45]

In an effort to gain further insight into the mechanism of the watery diarrhea, Kraft *et al.* examined the effects of purified gastrointestinal hormones and islet cell tumor extracts on active solute-solvent transport in a standardized rabbit gallbladder preparation.[47] Only natural secretin and extracts of the two original diarrheogenic tumors significantly inhibited mucosal-to-serosal transport of fluid. No other test substance had a similar effect on fluid absorption. Kraft concluded that "the watery diarrhea in the diarrheogenic syndrome results from not only the hypersecretion of bile and pancreatic juice but also the inhibition of active membrane transport of fluid and electrolytes." The similar inhibitory effect of pure secretin and extracts of diarrheogenic tumor on fluid transport was felt to add new evidence that the diarrheogenic hormone is secretin-like.

In the four years which have elapsed since the original suggestion that secretin is the diarrheogenic hormone, it cannot be said that there has been any avalanche of further case reports like that which followed the original communication on the ulcerogenic tumor. Dr. Wilfred Sircus, in a written communication dated January 4, 1969, stated that he had been able to extract a "pancreas-stimulating secretagogue" from pancreatic lesions in two patients with watery diarrhea, and that these extracts "behaved, in physiologic terms, as secretin. . . ." Professor J. Erik Jorpes (Fig. 70), in a separate communication dated March 28, 1969, stated that Mutt had found "substantial secretin-like activity" in a diarrheogenic tumor sent to them by Dr. Bengt Ihre (Fig. 71).

By July, 1969, Kraft, Tompkins, and Zollinger had been able to collect the case descriptions of 27 patients reported to have this syndrome from the available English and foreign literature.[57]

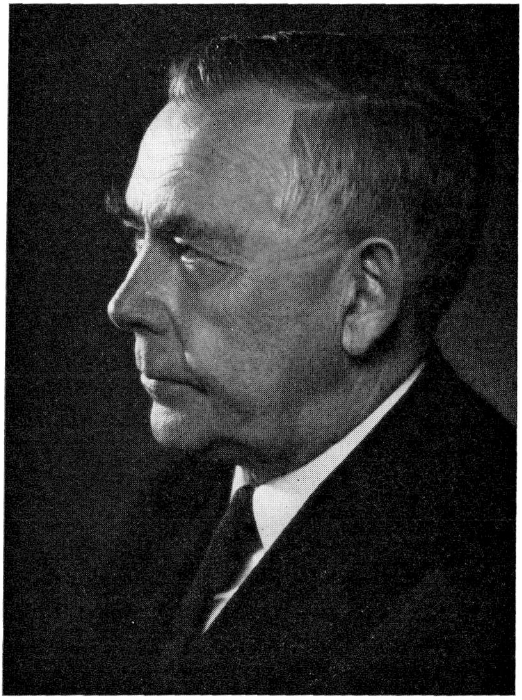

Figure 70. Dr. J. Erik Jorpes of the Karolinska Institutet of Stockholm; Sweden, whose method of extraction of secretin has been invaluable, both clinically and experimentally.

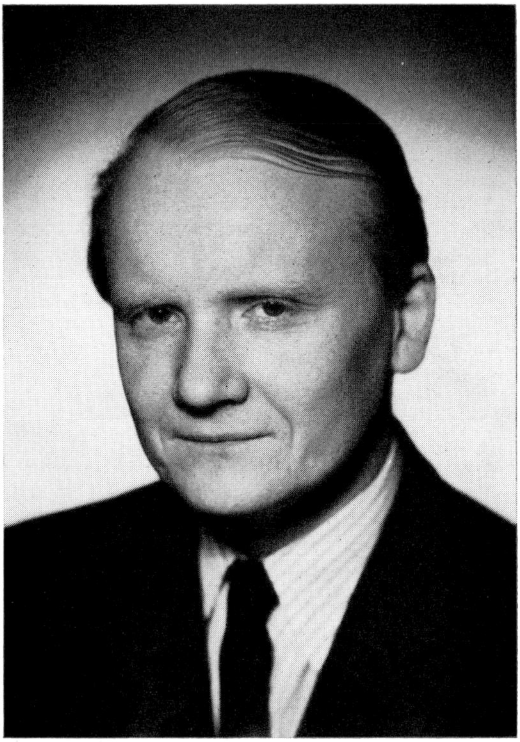

Figure 71. Dr. Viktor Mutt, a colleague of Professor Jorpes, extracted secretin-like activity from a diarrheogenic tumor.

This study was made in an effort to determine the outstanding clinical and laboratory findings and the most appropriate therapy for the "diarrheogenic syndrome." The major findings of this survey can be summarized under the following headings—

Series. The average age of the 17 female and 10 male patients was 44 at the time of diagnosis. The youngest patient was 19 and the oldest 67 years of age. A total of 15 patients met each of the established criteria (profuse watery diarrhea, hypokalemia, absence of gastric hypersecretion and a non-beta islet cell tumor) and were designated as *proved* cases. In the remaining 12 cases, the hypokalemia and absence of gastric hypersecretion was implied rather than measured. These patients were designated as *probable* cases.

Watery Diarrhea and Potassium Imbalance. The watery diarrhea averaged 5.8 L/day in 20 patients and was present an average of more than three years before the diagnosis of a pancreatic tumor was made. The serum potassium levels averaged 2.2 mEq/L during episodes of diarrhea. Despite intensive oral and parenteral replacement, stable correction was accomplished only after spontaneous remission of the diarrhea, excision of the tumor, or treatment with steroids.

Gastric Acid Studies. The absence of gastric hypersecretion is essential to the diagnosis of a diarrheogenic tumor. Of the 15 proved cases, 11 had basal achlorhydria, 2 had lower than normal acid values, and 2 were in the normal range. The achlorhydria was found, in various instances, to be reversible after histamine stimulation, complete tumor removal, or steroid medication. Five of the achlorhydric patients did not respond to histamine stimulation. Four of these were later found to have unresectable metastatic tumors.

Roentgenologic Studies. If large enough, the tumors may produce abnormalities on gastroduodenal roentgenograms, as in the senior author's case. Selective celiomesenteric arteriography was helpful in delineating tumor vascularity in one case, and in two additional cases, pancreas and liver scanning uncovered areas of tumor involvement.

Serum Calcium Alterations. Serum calcium levels were determined in 21 of the 27 cases, of which 16 (>90) had elevated levels. In two patients there was evidence of recurrent hypercalcemia despite removal of parathyroid adenomas or hyperplasia until either spontaneous cessation of the diarrhea or removal of the pancreatic tumor. Four additional patients with hypercalcemia who did not undergo neck exploration became normocalcemic after excision of the pancreatic tumors and control of the diarrhea. Kraft noted that these findings "suggested a parathormone-like effect of the non-beta islet cell tumor," or that "Alterations in magnesium balance might explain the elevated serum calcium levels . . . since hypomagnesemia is a known stimulus for parathormone release."

Glucose Tolerance Studies. Altered glucose metabolism was proven by glucose tolerance studies in about one third of the patients. In three patients, glucose tolerance tests after removal of the tumor returned to normal. It was theorized that this alteration in glucose might be related to the hypokalemia.

Preoperative Hormone Therapy. A total of eight patients were treated preoperatively with varying doses of corticosteroids. One patient who was later found to have a benign pancreatic tumor had definite improvement in the severe diarrhea. Two other patients with malignant pancreatic tumors experienced only temporary relief of the symptoms, while four were not improved.

Operative Findings and Pathology. A dilated gallbladder was observed in four cases, and analysis of the dilute bile from two of these showed the bile to be high in bicarbonate and chloride concentration such as occurs after the injection of secretin into animals. This secretin-like choleresis has been demonstrated for the third time in a recent personal case of the senior author. The duodenum and jejunum were observed to fill rapidly with bile and pancreatic secretions during the operations. Fifteen of the patients had malignant tumors and 25 per cent of them had spread at time of surgery. Twelve were found to have benign disease. Whether benign or malignant, the neoplasms were usually discrete and ranged in size from 1.5 to 7 cm in diameter. Of the 15 malignant tumors, three were multiple in the pancreas and 11 were metastatic.

Response to Treatment and Survival Rates. Operations ranging in extent from excision of the lesion to total pancreatectomy were performed in 14 patients. Five additional patients with malignant lesions underwent exploration and tumor biopsy alone. A negative exploration was carried out in one case and the diagnosis was not proven until postmortem examination. Removal of the primary tumor, whether malignant or benign, was successful in controlling the patients' diarrhea and improving their general condition in 11 patients. All patients treated surgically for benign tumors were alive and well with no recurrent symptoms when their cases were reported. Three of the seven patients having excision of malignant tumors were also known to be living and well when their cases were reported. The average length of survival for all patients with malignant disease was only one year. Postoperative corticosteroid therapy was used to control diarrhea in five patients whose neoplastic disease could not be totally extirpated. Temporary reduction in the stool volume was noted in all of these patients. Other forms of palliative treatment such as irradiation and chemotherapy have been associated with only short symptom-free remissions.

Findings similar to these were published in 1969 by John Verner in the proceedings of an international symposium on islet cell tumors which was held in Erlangen.[51] Verner said that "Glucagon assays need to be done on more tumors before one can completely exclude this hormone as playing a role in the clinical syndrome. The finding of hyperglycemia, . . . along with the earlier studies suggesting increased glucagon activity in patients with islet cell tumors again raises the possibility that increased glucagon secretion may occur in some of these patients." Further, in closing the discussion, he noted: "I go away with an increasing respect for the pancreas and gallbladder as potential organs for secretion. I just never thought of them in this syndrome." These words were spoken only three months after secretin was implicated in this syndrome.

Since that time, fewer than 20 additional cases have come to the attention of the senior author, including one personal case.

Patterson and Lopes *et al.*[58,59] both reported cases in which hypercalcemia appeared to occur in tandem. Patterson's patient, who had extensive metastatic disease, underwent a negative neck exploration with removal of two glands. Selenium scan subsequent to this and after the recurrence of diarrhea and hypercalcemia "suggested hyperfunctioning of the remaining left parathyroid gland." The patient expired and postmortem examination, if performed, was not reported. Patterson did note, however, that "The persistent hypercalcemia diverted us from the pancreas and delayed the diagnosis until the situation was not correctable." In discussing the etiology of this patient's diarrhea, he cited a normal secretin test as evidence that excessive pancreatic hypersecretion did not cause the diarrhea, though no reference was made to the previous papers.[46,50] The presence of a parathyroid adenoma in Lopes' case was not verified, but normocalcemia was *only* observed after removal of the islet cell tumor. Steroid therapy had no effect on the hypercalcemia. They postulated "the existence of a parathyroid-like hormone produced by the islet-cell adenoma."

Stoker and Wynn's[63] patient had flushing of the face and neck, recalling the observations of Chears,[15] Martini,[27] Murray,[18] Matsumoto,[34] Pabst,[48] Knappe,[33] and Lopes.[58] In all but Knappe's case, however, the urinary excretion of 5-hydroxyindoleacetic acid was normal; further, no hormone has yet been found to produce both flushing and diarrhea. It remains to be seen whether or not flushing is merely an incidental finding in the diarrheogenic syndrome. Acknowledging the senior author's evidence in favor of a secretin-like hormone, Stoker and Wynn raised the question, "What is not yet clear is how, in its further passage through the intestines, there is loss of normal water conservation together with electrolyte loss, the potassium loss being of greatest clinical significance." "The results in our patient show that the sodium and chloride content of the bowel fluid decreased, while that of potassium and bicarbonate increased, during the passage through the intestine. There is little evidence that a humoral mechanism exists for secretion from the wall of the small intestine."

Two companion papers by Gjone, Semb, and colleagues[55,61] were written about a 72-year-old man with the diarrheogenic syndrome who was treated in Oslo, Norway. A part of the primary pancreatic tumor was quickly frozen and transferred to New York Medical College where Rosenthal extracted the material according to methods developed there for separating gastrone. The extracts were assayed for "inhibitory activity" in Heidenhain pouch dogs. A different preparation was used to test the same extract for secretin activity. It was concluded that the tumor from this patient contained a "gastrone-like substance." Secretin activity could not be demonstrated in the extract when it was injected in a dose that showed gastric secretory inhibition. Gregory was unable to demonstrate gastrin in this tumor; likewise there was no glucagon-like effect of extracts on the blood glucose levels in dogs.

Sircus, Cleator, and colleagues[62] presented the clinical data of two women with pancreatic cholera. One had an islet cell adenoma; the other had islet cell hyperplasia. Hypercalcemia was a problem in the first case, and while a coexisting parathyroid adenoma was not excluded, the serum calcium returned to normal after removal of the tumor. Sircus suggested that it might be a "manifestation of tertiary hyperparathyroidism triggered by an initial low serum calcium induced by hyperglucagonemia."

Bioassays using cat, dog, and rat preparations were carried out on tumor extracts as well as plasma from these patients. The method of tumor extraction was essentially the same as that used by Zollinger *et al.* The extract of tumor from the first case caused an increase of the pancreatic output with the characteristics of a secretin-like response in both dog and cat. Plasma from the second case was found to contain both a pancreatic and a gastric secretagogue. No diarrhea occurred in any of the anesthetized animals during the assays. These workers concluded that:

> We have demonstrated the presence in the first case of a pancreatic secretagogue with secretin-like characteristics and with choleretic activity in terms of increased concentration of bilirubin in the bile. This choleretic character raises the possibility that the tumor elaborated small quantities of glucagon, but we had insufficient remaining tissue to allow us to examine this. That this patient also was episodically elaborating gastrin in excess is suggested by the clinical observations on her gastric secretion and by the plasma bioassays on the rat. . . . It seems probable that multiple factors are responsible for the profuse watery electrolyte-losing diarrhea, one of which may be an excessive production of secretin.

Grossman and his colleagues, in three separate communications, have challenged the concept that secretin is the diarrheogenic hormone. In a letter to the editor of *Lancet* on May 1, 1971, Barbezat and Grossman[65] wrote:

> We have found that glucagon stimulates the small intestine of dogs to secrete juice at remarkably high rates. In dogs with Thiry-Vella loops, intravenous infusion of 0.5μg/kg min of glucagon increased the flow of juice from basal levels of 2 to 3 ml/hr to peak levels of 11 ml/hr in jejunum and 17 ml/hr in ileum. The electrolyte composition of the juice was not greatly altered by glucagon. Both basal and glucagon juice were characteristic of the level of gut from which they came: low bicarbonate, high chloride in jejunum and high bicarbonate, low chloride and ileum. Synthetic secretin in equal doses did not reproduce the effect of glucagon. This finding raises

> the possibility that glucagon may be implicated in the severe watery diarrhea associated with certain non-beta pancreatic islet cell tumors.

These same authors, in a second letter dated May 15, 1971,[66] reported that they had been able to induce watery diarrhea in *intact* dogs by continuous intravenous infusions of a combination of glucagon (60μg/kg/hr) and pentagastrin (20μg/kg/hr.) This was repeatable in five different tests. The diarrhea began one to eight hours after starting the infusions and stopped promptly after the infusion of hormones was discontinued. They speculated that, "Perhaps pentagastrin potentiates the secretory effect of glucagon or impedes reabsorption. Another possibility is that pentagastrin, by relaxing the ileocecal sphincter, allows the profuse secretion from the small bowel to flow into the colon at a rate that exceeds colonic capacity."

Barbezat, in an essay submitted to the Southern California Society of Gastroenterology, enlarged upon these initial reports.[64] In this study, mongrel dogs were prepared surgically with Thiry-Vella loops of either the jejunum or the ileum. A Gregory cannula was inserted at each end of the loop and intestinal continuity was restored by end-to-end anastomosis. The effect of secretin, pentagastrin, and glucagon on the movement of water and electrolytes was then evaluated in a "systematic, controlled study." Barbezat found that glucagon increased the secretion of water, sodium, and chloride into the jejunum, while both pentagastrin and glucagon decreased the net absorption of sodium and water and increased the secretion of bicarbonate in the ileum. Secretin had no effect on either the jejunum or the ileum. In an effort to produce "cholera," intact dogs were given infusions of either glucagon alone, glucagon and the octapeptide of cholecystokinin, or glucagon and pentagastrin for periods of eight hours or until they developed diarrhea. Secretin was *not* used in this portion of the study. Glucagon alone had no noticeable effect. Glucagon plus the octapeptide of cholecystokinin produced explosive watery diarrhea. Glucagon combined with pentagastrin caused watery diarrhea on five different occasions. At doses that produced diarrhea in dogs, the glucagon in the mixture completely suppressed the stimulation of acid by pentagastrin, perhaps" . . .

mimicking the hypochlorhydria seen in patients with this syndrome."

In an attempt to determine the effect of specific gastrointestinal hormones on the human small intestine and further investigate the mechanism of watery diarrhea, Sanzenbacher *et al.*[68] utilized the triple-lumen tube perfusion technic in normal volunteers. The infusion part of the three lumen tube was positioned just distal to the ligament of Treitz (Fig. 72) and the test solution was infused at a constant rate of 10 cc/min. Intestinal contents are sampled at 15 and 45 cm distal to the point of infusion. In this way a 30 cm segment of proximal jejunum was studied and the secretions from the intestine proximal to the test segment were taken into account. Reflux or perfusate proximally was largely eliminated. The isotonic perfusion solution contained Na 145 mEq/L, Cl 140 mEq/L, K 5 mEq/L, bicarbonate 10 mEg/L, and PEG, 5 gm/L, as a non-absorbable maker. To facilitate measurement of the unidirectional movement of sodium. The proximal port was sampled by siphonage at a constant rate of 1 cc/min. As much fluid as could be obtained was collected from the distal port (Fig. 73).

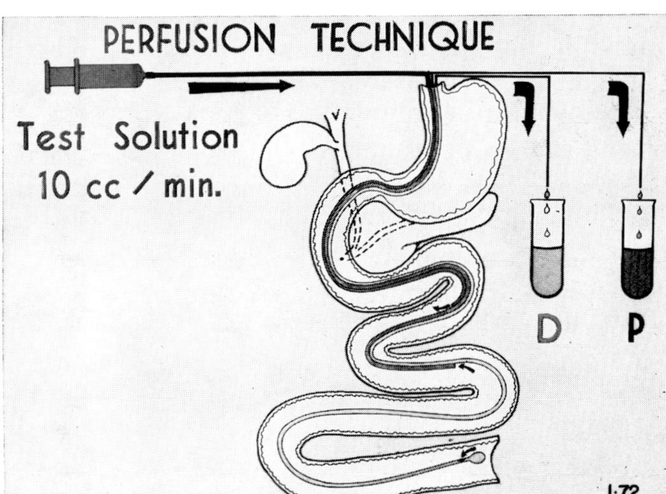

Figure 72. The triple lumen tube perfusion technic was used to investigate the mechanism of the watery diarrhea.

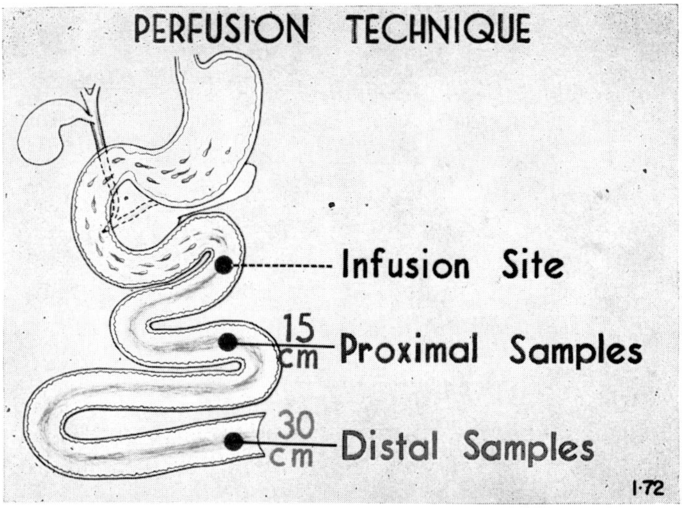

Figure 73. The infusion port of the tube was placed just distal to the ligament of Treitz and intestinal contents sampled 15 and 45 cm distal to the point of infusion.

During the control periods, the jejunum continuously *absorbed* water (1.68 ml/min), sodium 232μEq/min) and potassium 12.5μEq/min.). In contrast, a constant IV infusion of secretin (Jorpes, 4 U/kg/hr) produced an outpouring of fluid into the jejunal lumen. Water was *secreted* at a rate of 1/7 ml/min; sodium 290μEq/min, and potassium 9.6μEq/min (Fig. 74). Intravenous infusions of a combination of pentagastrin (Ayerst, 4μg/kg/hr) and glucagon (Lilly, 5μg/kg/hr) failed to cause secretion, but rather only a modest decrease in basal absorption: water 0.18 ml/min; sodium 18.9μEq/min, and potassium 2.6μEq/min (Fig. 75).

These data suggest that secretin causes an increase in jejunal succus entericus, rich in sodium and potassium, and add support to the concept that secretin, and not a gastrin-glucagon combination, is the diarrheogenic hormone associated with certain non-beta islet cell tumors of the pancreas.

The difference in results of these studies from those reported by Barbezat *et al.* may well be explained by the species difference.

Furthermore, in collaboration with Dr. T. M. Lin and Dr. R.

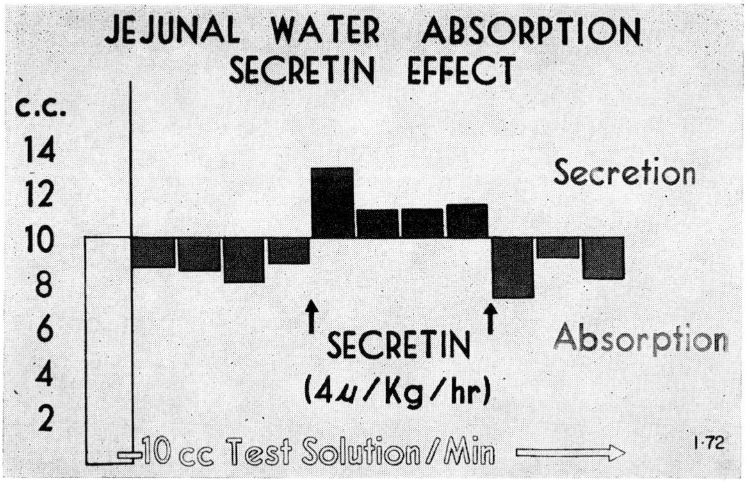

Figure 74. A constant intravenous infusion of Jorpes secretin produced an outpouring of fluid into the jejunal lumen.

Chance, extracts of two more recent diarrheogenic tumors have been prepared using a phosphoric-acid—alcohol method. A positive secretin-like response has been documented by bioassay for

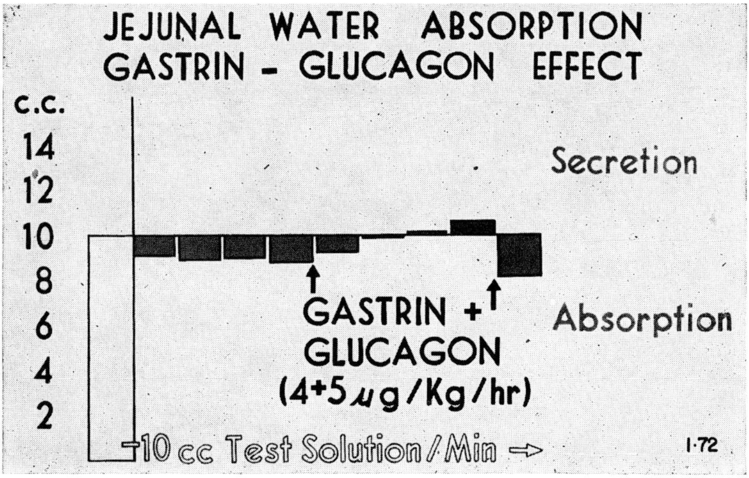

Figure 75. Intravenous infusions of a pentagastrin-glucagon combination caused only a modest decrease in basal absorption. They failed to cause secretion.

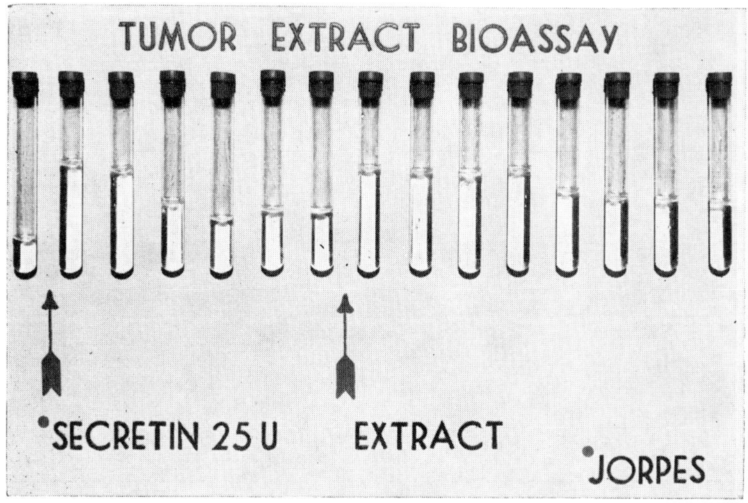

Figure 76. Two solid tumors have given similar pancreatic juice response in the Lin preparation with extractions made by a modification of the cold alcohol–phosphoric-acid method of Jackson.

both extracts (Fig. 76). In addition to an increase in pancreatic juice, rich in bicarbonate, IV infusion of the extracts also produced inhibition of gastric acid secretion and an increase in bile flow.

The presence of gastrin, glucagon and insulin in the extracts has been excluded by radioimmunoassay for the respective peptides.

It is hoped that amino acid sequence of these tumor extracts will be forthcoming shortly as the clinching evidence supporting secretin, the first hormone described in 1903.

It would be sheer folly not to predict that many more significant polypeptides, some with quite similar actions, will be extracted from the pancreas as well as the remainder of the gastrointestinal tract. As they are discovered and their relationship to clinical syndromes developed, the advances in immunoassays will assure earlier and more specific diagnosis than in the past. Gastrin and secretin have now been associated with definite clinical syndromes. They provide a rich field for further clinical and research investigation. The true value of Beaumont's original contribution is yet to be fully realized.

REFERENCES

1937

1. Agren, E., and Lagerlof, H.: The biliary response to the secretin test. *Acta Med Scand, 92:*359, 1937.

1947

2. Gordon, B. S., and Olivetti, R. G.: Carcinoma of the islets of Langerhans. *Gastroenterology, 9:*409, 1947.

1950

3. Brown, C. H., Neville, W. E., and Hazard, J. B.: Islet-cell adenoma, without hypoglycemia, causing duodenal obstruction. *Surgery, 27:* 616, 1950.

1951

4. Lowry, O. H., Rosebrough, N. J., Farr, A. L., and Randall, R. J.: Protein measurement with the folin phenol reagent. *J Biol Chem, 193:*265, 1951.
5. Natelson, S.: Estimation of sodium potassium, chloride, protein, hematocrit value, sugar, urea and non-protein nitrogen in fingertip blood. Construction of ultramicro pipets. A practical microgastrometer for estimation of carbon dioxide. *Am J Clin Path, 21:*1153, 1951.

1952

6. Forty, F., and Barrett, G. M.: Peptic ulceration of the third part of the duodenum associated with islet-cell tumors of the pancreas. Brit *J Surg, 40:*60, 1952–53.

1954

7. Moldawer, M. P., Nardi, G. L., and Raker, J. W.: Concomitance of multiple adenomas of the parathyroids and pancreatic islets with tumor of the pituitary: A syndrome with familial incidence. *Am J Med Sci, 228:*190, 1954.

1955

8. Zollinger, R. M., and Ellison, E. H.: Primary peptic ulcerations of the jejunum associated with islet cell tumors of the pancreas. *Ann Surg, 142:*709, 1955.

1956

9. Code, C. F.: Quantitative determination of histamine. In Glick, D. (Ed.): *Methods of Biochemical Analysis.* New York: Interscience Publishers, Vol. 3, p. 49, 1956.

1957

10. Greenlee, H. B., Longhi, E. H., Guerrero, J., *et al.:* Inhibitory effect of pancreatic secretin on gastrin secretion. *Am J Physiol, 190:*396, 1957.
11. Priest, W. M., and Alexander, M. K.: Islet-cell tumor of the pancreas

with peptic ulceration, diarrhea, and hypokalemia. *Lancet, 2:*1145, 1957.

1958

12. Verner, J. V., and Morrison, A. B.: Islet cell tumor and a syndrome of refractory watery diarrhea and hypokalemia. *Am J Med, 25:*374, 1958.

1959

13. Caraway, W. T.: A stable starch substrate for the determination of amylase in serum and other body fluids. *Am J Clin Path, 32:*97, 1959.

1960

14. Charles, B., and Cochran, W. A.: Islet cell tumor of the pancreas with chronic diarrhea and hypokalemia—A recently recognized syndrome. *Canad Med Ass J, 82:*579, 1960.
15. Chears, W. C., Thompson, J. E., Hutcheson, J. B., and Patterson, C. O.: Pancreatic islet tumor with severe diarrhea. *Am J Med, 24:*529, 1960.
16. Gregory, R. A., Tracy, H. J., French, J. M., *et al.:* Extraction of a gastrin-like substance from a pancreatic tumor in a case of Zollinger-Ellison syndrome. *Lancet, 1:*1045, 1960.

1961

17. Parkins, R. A.: Severe watery diarrhea and potassium depletion associated with an islet-cell tumor of the pancreas. *Brit Med J, 2:*356, 1961.
18. Murray, J. S., Paton, R. R., and Pope, C. E.: Pancreatic tumor associated with flushing and diarrhea. *New Eng J Med, 264:*436, 1961.
19. Telling, M., and Smiddy, F. G.: Islet tumors of the pancreas with intractable diarrhea. *Gut, 2:*12, 1961.

1962

20. Espiner, E. A., and Beaven, D. W.: Non-specific islet-cell tumor of the pancreas with diarrhea. *Quart J Med, 124:*447, 1962.
21. Lin, T. M., and Alphin, R. S.: Comparative bioassay of secretin and pancreozymin in rats and dogs. *Am J Physiol, 203:*926, 1962.

1963

22. Bruggisser, R., and Merki, W.: Islet cell tumor of the pancreas with intractable diarrhea. *Helvet Med Acta, 4:*540, 1963.

1964

23. Boulet, P., Barjon, P., Prioton, J. B., *et al.:* Diarrhee chronique avec depletion potassique d'origine pancreatique. Les limits due syndrom de Verner et Morrison. *J Rean Med Chir,* p. 24, 1964. (Quoted by Goulon, M., *et al*[17]).
24. Brown, C. H., and Crile, G.: Pancreatic adenoma with intractable diarrhea, hypokalemia, and hypercalcemia. *JAMA, 190:*142, 1964.

25. Deleu, J., Tytgat, H., and Van Goidsenhoven, G. E.: Diarrhea associated with pancreatic islet-cell tumors. *Am J Dig Dis, 9:*97, 1964.
26. Hindle, W., McBrien, D. J., and Creamer, B.: Watery diarrhea and islet cell tumor. *Gut, 5:*359, 1964.
27. Martini, G. A., Strohmeyer, G., Haug, P., and Gusek, W.: Islet cell adenoma of the pancreas with urticarial exanthem, diarrhea as well as loss of potassium and protein by way of the intestine. *Deutsch Med Wochenschr, 89:*313, 1964.

1965

28. Smith, R.: The Zollinger-Ellison syndrome. *Ann Roy Coll Surg (Eng), 37:*160, 1965.
29. Wheeler, H. O.: Inorganic ions in bile. In Taylor, W. (Ed.): *The Biliary System.* Philadelphia: F. A. Davis, 481, 1965.

1966

30. Bodanszky, M., von Saltza, M., Levine, S. D., *et al:* Synthesis of a heptacosapeptide amide with the hormonal activity of secretin. *Chem Industr, 42:*1757, 1966.
31. Gardner, J. D., and Cerda, J. J.: In vitro inhibition f intestinal fluid and electrolyte transfer by a non-beta islet cell tumor. *Proc Exp Biol Med, 123:*361, 1966.
32. Goulon, M., *et al.:* Aqueous diarrhea and hypokalemia associated with a non-insulinogenic Langerhans tumor. A case of immediate and definite cure of the diarrhea by excision of the tumor. *Soc Med Hop Paris, 117:*623, 1966.
33. Knappe, G., Flemming, F., H. Strobbe, H., and Wendt, F.: Pancreatic islet cell adenoma with the triad of diarrhea, hypokalemia and hyperglycemia. *Deutsch Med Wachenschr, 91:*1224, 1966.
34. Matsumoto, K. K., Peter, J. B., Schultze, R. G., *et al.:* Watery diarrhea and hypokalemia associated with pancreatic islet cell adenoma. *Gastroenterology, 50:*231, 1966.
35. Zaterka, S., and Grossman, M. I.: The effect of gastrin and histamine on secretion of bile. *Gastroenterology, 50:*500, 1966.
36. Zenker, R., Forell, M. M., and Erpenbeck, R.: A rare syndrome produced by a pancreas adenoma. *Deutsch Med Wochenschr, 91:*634, 1966.

1967

37. DaCruz, G. M., Gardner, J. V., and Peskin, G. W.: Influence of gastrointestinal tumors on intestinal absorption. *Surg Forum, 18:*336, 1967.
38. Gardner, J. J., Peskin, G. W., Cerda, J. J., and Brooks, F. P.: Alterations of in vitro fluid and electrolyte absorption by gastrointestinal hormones. *Am J Surg, 113:*57, 1967.
39. Kofstad, J., Froyshov, I., Gjone, E., and Blix, S.: Pancreatic tumor with intractable watery diarrhea, hypokalemia and hypercalcemia electrolyte balance studies. *Scand J Gastroenterol, 2:*246, 1967.

40. Marks, I. N., Bank, S., and Louw, J. H.: Islet cell tumor of the pancreas with reversible watery diarrhea and achlorhydria. *Gastroenterology, 52:*695, 1967.
41. Umeyama, K., Nakayama, K., and Koike, M.: Case of non-functioning cancer of the islands of Langerhans with chronic diarrhea as the chief complaint. *Jap J Clin Med, 25:*337, 1967.

1968

42. Hess, W.: Diarrhea with hypokalemia, prediabetes and subacidity. A new syndrome in hyperfuction of the insular apparatus. *Helv Chir Acta, 35:*87, 1968.
43. Johansen, P. G., Hadorn, B., and Anderson, D. M.: Effect of secretin on human rectal mucosa in vivo. *Nature, 217:*468, 1968.
44. Scott, H. W., in discussion of Zollinger, R. M., Tompkins, R. K., Amerson, J. R., *et al.:* Identification of the diarrheogenic hormone associated with non-beta islet cell tumors of the pancreas. *Ann Surg, 168:*520, 1968.
45. Wormsley, K. G.: Response to secretin in man. *Gastroenterology, 54:*197, 1968.
46. Zollinger, R. M., Tompkins, R. K., Amerson, J. R., et al.: Identification of the diarrheogenic hormone associated with non-beta islet cell tumors of the pancreas. *Ann Surg, 168:*502, 1968.

1969

47. Kraft, A. R., Tompkins, R. K., Endahl, G. L., *et al.:* Alteration in membrane transport produced by diarrheogenic non-beta islet cell tumors of the pancreas. *Surg Forum, 20:*338, 1969.
48. Pabst, K., et al.: Contribution on the clinical picture of the Verner-Morrison syndrome. *Dsch Med Wochenshr, 94:*9, 1969.
49. Pabst, K., Kummerle, F., and Hennekeuser, H. H.: The clinical picture of the Verner-Morrison syndrome. Dsch Med *Wochenshr, 1:*9, 1969.
50. Tompkins, R. K., Kraft, A. R., and Zollinger, R. M.: Secretin-like choleresis produced by a diarrheogenic non-beta islet cell tumor of the pancreas. *Surgery, 66:*131, 1969.
51. Verner, J. V.: Clinical syndromes with non-insulin-producing tumors of the pancreatic islets. In Demling, L., and Ottenjann, R. (Eds.): *Non-Insulin-Producing Tumors of the Pancreas: Modern Aspects on Zollinger-Ellison Syndrome and Gastrin.* Stuttgart: Georg Thieme Verlag, 1969.

1970

52. Brunt, P. W., *et al.:* Secretory tumors of pancreas. Pancreatic tumor associated with life-threatening diarrhea. *J Roy Coll Surg Edinb, 15:*200, 1970.
53. Cerda, J. J., Raffensperger, E. C., and Rawnsley, H. M.: Cholera-like syndrome and pancreatic islet cell tumors. *Med Clin N Am, 54:*567, 1970.

54. Cleator, J. G. M., Thomson, C. G., Sircus, W., *et al.:* Bio-assay evidence of abnormal secretin-like and gastrin-like activity in tumor and blood in cases of 'choleraic diarrhoea.' *Gut, 11:*206, 1970.
55. Gjone, E., Fretheim, B., Nordoy, A., *et al.:* Intractable watery diarrhea, hypokalemia, and achlorhydria associated with pancreatic tumor containing secretory inhibitor. *Scand J Gastroent, 5:*401, 1970.
56. Koenen-Schmahling, R., *et al.:* Verner-Morrison syndrome: A case report. *Munchen Med Wachenshr, 112:*98, 1970.
57. Kraft, A. R., Tompkins, R. K., and Zollinger, R. M.: Recognition and management of the diarrheal syndrome caused by non-beta islet cell tumors of the pancreas. *Am J Surg, 119:*163, 1970.
58. Lopes, Virginia M., Reis, D. R., and Cunha, Amelia, B.: Islet-cell adenoma of the pancreas with reversible watery diarrhea and hypokalemia. *Am J Gastroent, 53:*17, 1970.
59. Patterson, M.: The diagnosis of the Zollinger-Ellison syndrome. *Am J Gastroent, 54:*470, 1970.
60. Rambaud, J. C., Mignon, F., Hautefeuille, P., et al.: Verner-Morrison syndrome with non-tumoral form. A Case. *Rev Med Chir Mal Foie, 45:*261, 1970.
61. Semb, L. S., Gjone, E., and Rosenthal, W. S.: Bioassay for gastric secretory inhibitor in extract of pancreatic tumor from patient with WDHA-syndrome. *Scand J Gastroent, 5:*409, 1970.
62. Sircus, W., Brunt, P. W., Walker, R. J., *et al.:* Two cases of 'pancreatic cholera' with features of peptide-secreting adenomatosis of the pancreas. *Gut, 11:*197, 1970.
63. Stoker, D. J., and Wynn, V.: Pancreatic islet cell tumor with watery diarrhea and hypokalemia. *Gut, 11:*911, 1970.

1971

64. Barbezat, G. O.: Experimental "cholera" in the dog induced by gastro-intestinal hormones.
65. Barbezat, G. O., and Grossman, M. I.: Glucagon stimulates intestinal secretion. *Lancet, I:*918, 1971.
66. Barbezat, G. O., and Grossman, M. I.: Cholera-like diarrhea induced by glucagon plus gastrin. *Lancet, I:*1025, 1971.
67. Rosenthal, W. S.: Glucagon stimulation of intestinal secretion: Does it cause watery diarrhea? *Lancet, II:*497, 1971.

1972

68. Sanzenbacher, L. J., Mekhjian, H. S., King, D. R., et al.: Studies on the potential role of secretin in the islet cell tumor diarrheogenic syndrome. *Ann Surg, 176:*3, Sept. 1972.

Section III

THE LIFE AND ACCOMPLISHMENTS OF WILLIAM BEAUMONT

America's Pioneer Surgeon-Scientist

The observations recorded in this monograph concerning the hormonal effects of certain islet cell tumors of the pancreas might not have been possible without the original observations by Dr. William Beaumont. By initiating gastrointestinal physiologic research, he stimulated physiologists, clinicians, and many others to observe the interesting challenge of digestion and the factors which influence the secretion of hydrochloric acid. The islet cell tumors under discussion in this monograph are the first examples of a pancreatic source being responsible for a marked effect on the secretion of hydrochloric acid producing two definite clinical syndromes.

The life of William Beaumont began November 21, 1785, in Lebanon, Connecticut. His travels ended 68 years later on April 25, 1853, in St. Louis, where he had sustained a head injury after falling on ice-covered steps while returning home from a professional call (Color Plate 1).

Young William Beaumont, the third of nine children, represented the sixth generation of Beaumonts in America. Little is known of his early childhood which was spent on the farm owned by his father, Samuel. A life of soil tilling and churchgoing apparently did not satisfy Beaumont and in the winter of 1806-07, shortly after his twenty-first birthday, he left for the North country. He settled in the village of Champlain, New York, where his Uncle William* lived, and remained here for the next three years, teaching school, tending store, and saving money for his further education in medicine.

---

* Beaumont's great, great grandfather, Pliny Moore, was the first settler of Champlain, New York.

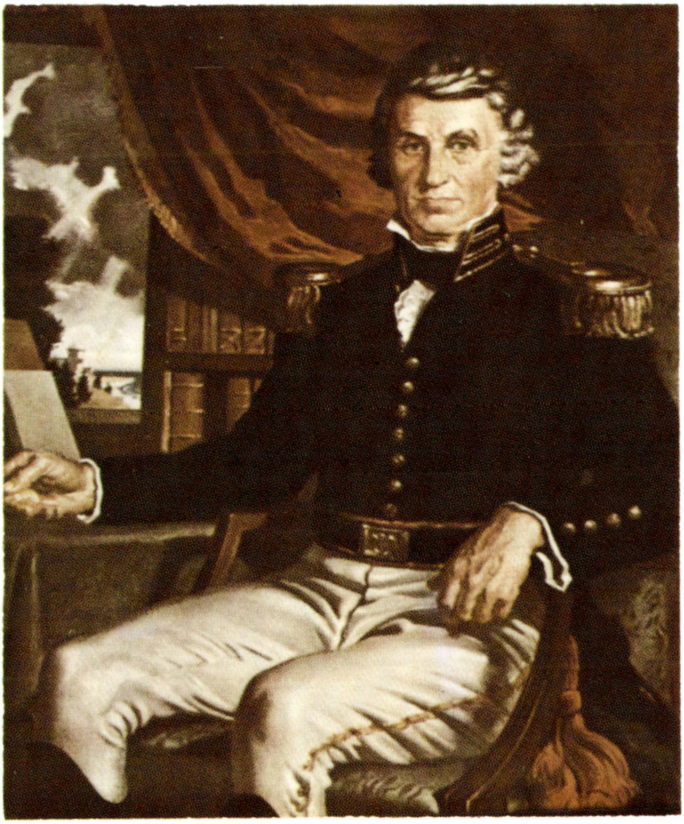

Color Plate 1. A painted photograph of William Beaumont, hanging in the Beaumont Medical Library of Yale University School of Medicine.

A medical apprentice in the early 1800's was both student and employee. His duties ranged from sweeping floors and washing bottles to mixing pills and powders and assisting at operations. As if in a perpetual clinic, he learned something of symptoms, diagnosis, and treatment, as well as prescription writing and basic sickroom procedures. In the words of Harvey Cushing,[3] "The only thing he omitted was to prepare himself in the methods of experimental research, but then where could such preparation be had?" In these days of streamlined curricula, from premedical to advanced postgraduate programs, we can well take consolation in the background of William Beaumont, who had no college training or research experience, save for a two-year apprenticeship.

The man of his choice for a preceptor in medical education was Dr. Benjamin Chandler of St. Albans, Vermont, who is said to have played a considerable part in the development of Beaumont's most outstanding characteristics in later life: a trained memory, keen powers of observation, and the habit of thinking and acting logically combined with a tendency to be a compulsive diarist.

Beaumont was licensed to practice medicine on the second Tuesday of June, 1812, by the Third Medical Society of Vermont. In September, 1812, he left Dr. Chandler and joined the Army as Assistant Surgeon. Beaumont saw a great deal of action during the war of 1812, and was cited by name in a group of five medical officers "who, for their particular services . . . merit the applause of the country." His military experiences provided a background for the subsequent care of his world-famous patient, Alexis St. Martin.

After the war, Beaumont and Dr. G. Senger (another Army surgeon) in December, 1815, commenced the practice of "physic and surgery" and also opened a store in Plattsburg, New York, to dispense "drugs, medicines, dye, woods, etc." This experience, coupled with his fine war record, won him unqualified respect as a physician and surgeon. It was also during this period that he courted, with eventual success, Mrs. Deborah Platt (nee Green), the widowed daughter of Israel Green. Beaumont's mind, however, was constantly plagued by thoughts of military service. One of his former comrades, Dr. Joseph Lovell, was appointed first Surgeon-General of the United States Army in 1818 (Fig. 77). He and Beaumont had met and became close friends while in a garrison hospital in Oswego, New York, during the war. As months passed, posts in the newly organized United States Army Medical Corps became more attractive, and Beaumont applied for readmission to the service.

He was immediately ordered to the fort of Mackinac Island, whereupon he quit his practice, settled his accounts, and recommended to the people of Clinton Township that they give their patronage to his cousin, Dr. Samuel Beaumont.

He set out for Michigan on May 6, 1820. The roads and waterways of that time were long and wandering, and they took him by post and stagecoach, by river and canal boat. On the evening

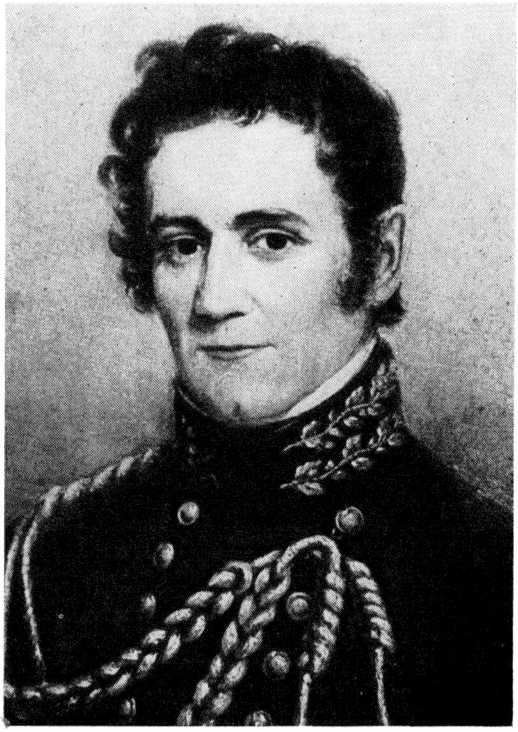

Figure 77. Brigadier-General Joseph Lovell, the first Surgeon General of the United States Army, strongly supported the work of Beaumont and provided opportunities for him to verify his early experiments.

of June 16, 41 days after he left Plattsburgh, Beaumont reported to Major General Alexander Macomb, who had been his commanding officer at the Battle of Plattsburgh. He was the only physician within 300 miles.

Soon after his arrival, Beaumont wrote to Surgeon-General Lovell for permission to engage in private practice; perhaps it was he who introduced the concept of "moonlighting."[2] Lovell replied: "The Secretary of War has no objection to your giving your professional services to the sick of Mackinac, provided it does not interfere with your official duties. They cannot, however, be furnished from the public chest."

Though busy with work he liked at Mackinac, Beaumont could not reconcile himself to separation from Deborah Platt. He requested and was granted a furlough long enough to permit a trip east, a wedding, and the return trip with his bride (Fig. 78).

ST. MARTIN'S INJURY AND CONVALESCENCE, 1822-25

Early in June of 1822, Indians and voyageurs were returning to Mackinac from Canada with the results of their winter's catch.

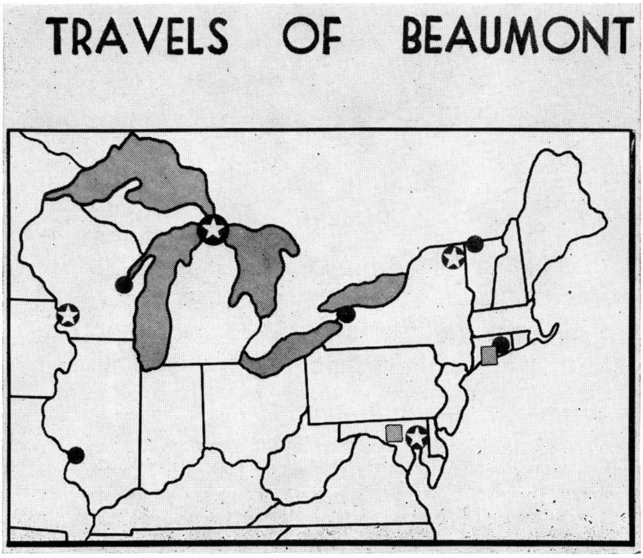

Figure 78. Beaumont's professional life was largely along the frontiers. Stars and squares indicate locations of experimental observations.

The little village had awaken from its long sleep and the beach was crowded again with tents and wigwams of about 3,000 men in the employ of the American Fur Company. One, Alexis St. Martin, was among this group.

A shotgun was accidentally discharged in the American Fur Company retail store on the bright spring morning of June 16, 1822, and the young voyageur Alexis St. Martin dropped to the floor with a cavity in his left upper abdomen that would have admitted a man's fist. He proved to be a young French Canadian, about 28 years of age,* who had recently come down from Montreal.

Gordon S. Hubbard was an eyewitness of this accident and apparently the only one who left any written statement concerning the affair: "The muzzle was not over three feet from him—I think not more than two. The wadding entered as well as pieces of clothing, his shirt took fire; he fell, and we supposed, dead."

Within 15 to 20 minutes, by his own estimate, Beaumont arrived on the scene. He knew this was more than a mere perforating wound and described it as an "altogether appalling and hopeless case." Beaumont left the store with this account: "The man can't live thirty-six hours. I will come to see him by-and-by." According to Hubbard, Beaumont visited St. Martin two or three hours after the first call. The next day he brought instruments to remove more shots and bits of clothing and to cut off ragged edges of the wound. For the next 11 years or so, the lives of William Beaumont and Alexis St. Martin were to be inexorably entwined.

At the time of this accident, Beaumont had other matters of importance on his mind. In addition to this emergency, plus the regular duties at the hospital, his wife, Deborah, was expecting shortly the birth of their first child. Sarah Beaumont was born safely in the family living quarters on June 18 while St. Martin lay fighting for his life at the nearby hospital. For a distracting

* The question of St. Martin's age has long been a matter of controversy. Not until the 1930's were parish records discovered which showed that St. Martin was born on April 18, 1794, and baptized in the Roman Catholic faith at Berthier in lower Quebec. Parish records also established that the young man's family name was not originally St. Martin. He was descended from a French line bearing the surname Bidegan, but his forebearers, on their arrival in Canada, added the St. Martin, and the boy was christened Alexis Bidegan, dit St. Martin.

interval of 48 hours, Beaumont rushed back and forth from one patient to the other. Then with mother and daughter doing well and St. Martin out of immediate danger, he settled into a new routine that was not seriously disturbed for nearly two years. Day after day, for more than two years, Beaumont recorded every detail of his progress. This record is considered a model of thoroughness and accuracy and is reprinted in whole or in part in several available Beaumont biographies.[5,6,7] About five days after the accident, a sloughing of muscle and skin took place in and around the wound, giving a plain view of the perforation into the stomach and exposing a part of the lung. A violent fever continued for 10 days, after which the whole surface of the wound assumed a healthy appearance. Beaumont recorded that for 17 days, all that entered St. Martin's stomach by the esophagus soon passed out through the wound. A few days later, firm dressing were applied and the contents of the stomach retained. Beaumont wrote "not even the slightest nausea was manifest during the whole time: and after the fourth week the appetite became good, digestion regular . . . and all the functions of the system perfect and healthy."

During the fifth week, the contraction of the external wound and the formation of scar tissue started. The stomach became more firmly attached to the chest wall, *"but showed not the least disposition to close its orifice"* (Fig. 79). Thus, instead of falling back into the cavity of the abdomen to its natural position, the prolapsed portion of the stomach remained in contact with the external wound, affording a free passage out, and fair opportunity to apply protective dressings. Hubbard[5] suggested that St. Martin's wound was purposely left open; such was not the case. Beaumont even proposed freshening the wound edges and closing it with sutures, but St. Martin would not consent to the operation.

Beaumont sent a complete report of St. Martin's case to Surgeon-General Lovell for approval and correction in the fall of 1824. The article appeared in the *Philadelphia Medical Recorder* in January, 1825, but through an oversight was published as "A Case of Wounded Stomach, by Joseph Lovell, M.D., Surgeon-General, U.S.A" (Fig. 80). Toward the end of the year, a correction of the authorship was inserted in the Journal. By this time,

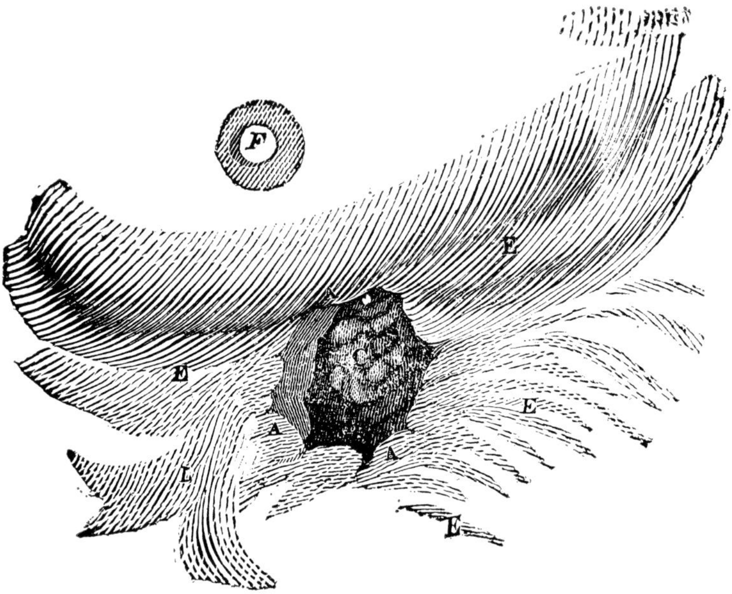

Figure 79. The appearance of the gastrostomy in Alexis St. Martin from a woodcut in the original edition of Beaumont's "Experiments and Observations."

Beaumont had obviously crystallized the idea of experimenting on St. Martin, for in the conclusion to this report, he wrote:

> This case affords a most excellent opportunity of experimenting upon the gastric fluids, and the process of digestion. It would give no pain, nor cause the least uneasiness, to extract a gill of fluid every two

BEAUMONT'S EXPERIMENTS (238)*

ST. MARTIN'S INJURY *	**MACKINAC**	**1822**
Experiments		
4 *	**Mackinac**	**1825**
56	**Prairie due Chien**	**1829-31**
116	**Plattsburgh**	**1832**
	Washington, D.C.	**1833**
62	**Plattsbourgh**	**1833**

Figure 80. The titles of the publications by William Beaumont reporting the initial four experiments and the subsequent 238 experiments on Alexis St. Martin.

or three days; for it frequently flows out spontaneously in considerable quantities; and one might introduce various digestible substances into the stomach, and easily examine them during the whole process of digestion. I may, therefore, be able hereafter to give some interesting experiments on these subjects.

As Sir William Osler was to say, many years later, "The man and the opportunity had met."[5]

Beaumont now began to feel keenly his complete isolation and realized the great difficulties that confronted him in conducting experiments under the conditions at Mackinac. In June, 1825, he was ordered to Fort Niagara; St. Martin went with him. He then took St. Martin to Burlington and Plattsburgh (Fig. 78). Without obtaining Beaumont's consent, St. Martin fled to Canada.

FIRST SERIES OF EXPERIMENTS, AUGUST 1-8, 1825.

Beaumont then decided to publish the results of the few observations he had made and sent a series of experiments to the *Philadelphia Medical Recorder.* They were published in January, 1826 ("Further Experiments on the Case of Alexis San Martin, 9 (33)94, 1826"), as a supplement to the previous case reported under Lovell's name. This series of experiments numbered four.[5] Beaumont noted the length of time required for the digestion of various articles of food suspended in the stomach by a silk string. He determined the "natural warmth" of the stomach and compared the length of time of digestion of certain articles in the stomach and in vials containing gastric juice at body temperature, agitated from time to time to stimulate gastric peristalsis. Beaumont found that digestion took place more rapidly in the stomach than in the vials after the first half hour and that some meats digested more slowly than others because the texture was closer. These incomplete experiments assured him that the old theories of maceration and putrefaction were not sufficient to explain the processes that he had observed and that the gastric juice possessed innate solvent powers (Fig. 81).

BEAUMONT IN MICHIGAN TERRITORY, 1826-29

Beaumont was now transferred to Fort Howard at Green Bay in Wisconsin, having again received permission to "moonlight"

PUBLICATIONS
"A Case of Wounded Stomach"
Lovell, Med. Rec., 1825
"Further Experiments on the Case
of San Martin"
Beaumont, Med. Rec., 1826
"EXPERIMENTS & OBSERVATIONS
ON THE GASTRIC JUICE. . . . ."
Beaumont, Plattsburgh, 1833

Figure 81. The number and locations of the experiments carried out by Beaumont totaled 238 experiments over a period of approximately 11 years.

with a civilian practice. Much the same conditions prevailed here as in Mackinac. In two years, Beaumont built up a reputation as a practitioner and surgeon and also acquired considerable property.

In January of 1828, nearly 2½ years after his unceremonious departure, Beaumont received news of St. Martin. W. W. Matthews of the American Fur Company wrote Beaumont that he had found St. Martin and that he was married and living 12 miles from Berthier in Canada. In the meantime, Beaumont had received orders to join the Fifth Regiment at Fort Crawford (Prairie du Chien) also in the Michigan territory. He arrived there on August 10, 1826.

Almost two years elapsed since receiving the news of St. Martin's whereabouts, and in the meantime, the officers of the fur company made every effort to bring him back to Beaumont. Without the efforts of Ramsey Crooks, W. W. Matthews, and William Morrison, St. Martin's case would have been lost to science. They transported St. Martin, his wife, and their two children from Lower Canada to Fort Crawford, a distance of nearly 2,000 miles, in August, 1829. His stomach and side were in similar condition as when he left Beaumont in 1825. The aperture was open and his health good.

SECOND SERIES OF EXPERIMENTS, DECEMBER 6, 1829 TO APRIL 9, 1831

The second series of experiments were begun on December 6, 1829, and continued until April 9, 1831, while Beaumont and St.

Martin were in Fort Crawford. There was a total of 56 experiments (Fig. 81). In summing up the 56 experiments, Beaumont said: "The preceding experiments, I think, plainly demonstrate the solvent properties of the gastric juice." During this time, St. Martin performed the duties of a common servant, with little or no suffering or inconvenience from his wound.

THIRD SERIES OF EXPERIMENTS, DECEMBER 1, 1832 TO MARCH 1, 1833

In September, 1832, Beaumont returned to Plattsburgh via St. Louis, at which time St. Martin appeared on the scene. He endeavored unsuccessfully to force the loyalty of St. Martin to him through a legal document and then decided to spend six months' furlough with St. Martin in Washington, D.C., where he would have access to literature on the physiology of digestion. Dr. Lovell was able to render much assistance to him and did freely. According to Osler, Beaumont tried to induce Surgeon-General Lovell to undertake the arrangement for the observations, but Lovell insisted that Beaumont should do the work himself. In addition, through Lovell, St. Martin, although a Canadian citizen, was made sergeant of a detachment of orderlies in the War De-

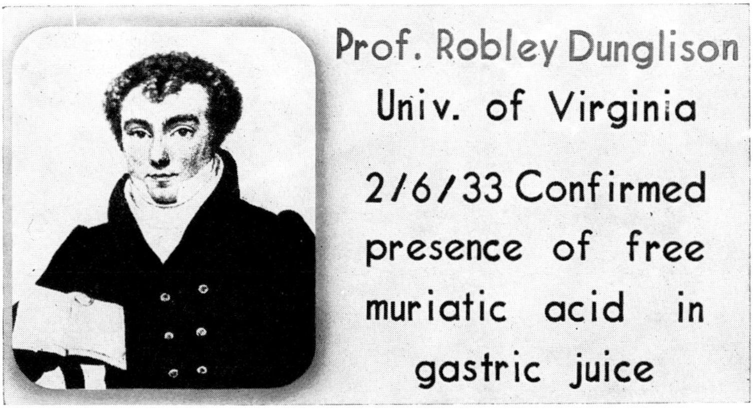

Figure 82. Professor Robley Dunglison, the first fulltime Professor of Medicine in the United States at the University of Virginia and the personal physician to Thomas Jefferson, confirmed for Beaumont the presence of free muriatic acid in gastric juice.

partment. His stipend was $12.00 per month with a monthly allowance of $2.50 for clothing and 10 cents per day for subsistence.

Beaumont started on his third series of experiments and between December 1, 1832, and March 1, 1833, recorded 116 observations, some of which merely confirmed what he had done before (Fig. 81).

While in the midst of these researchers, Beaumont successfully enlisted the assistance of two of America's leading scientists, Robley Dunglison, first full-time Professor of Medicine in this country and physician to Thomas Jefferson and Professor of Physiology in the Medical Department of the University of Virginia (Fig. 82), and Professor Benjamin Silliman of Yale (Fig. 83).

Dunglison traveled to Washington to confer with Beaumont, who most wanted a careful chemical analysis to determine the solvent ingredients of gastric juice. In a letter to Beaumont, dated February 6, 1833, Dunglison said: ". . . we have found it to con-

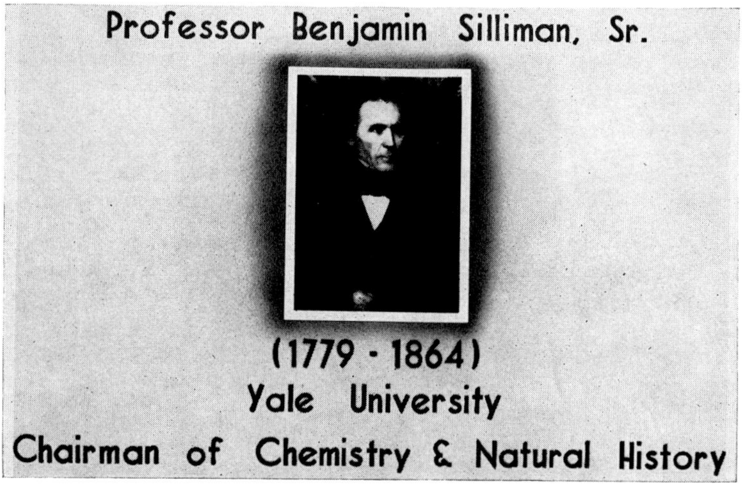

Figure 83. Dr. Benjamin Silliman Sr., Professor of Chemistry and Natural History at Yale University, was perhaps the most famous chemist of his day. He founded the American Journal of Science and was instrumental in having Beaumont send some of the gastric juice to Professor Berzelius of Stockholm.

tain free muriatic and acetic acid, phosphates and muriates, with bases of potassium, soda, magnesia and lime, and an animal matter soluble in cold water, but insoluble in hot. We were satisfied, you will recollect, in Washington that free muriatic acid was present, but I had no conception it existed in the amount met with in our experiments here."

In March of 1833, Beaumont was ordered to New York City, and by means of a special furlough, St. Martin was allowed to accompany him on this trip. Shortly after his arrival there, a letter came from Dunglison, which said that far from being able to "fix with certainty . . . the other ingredients," he had arrived at the conclusions "that the precise constituents of the gastric juice may never be accurately determined." It remained for Schwann, in 1833, to announce the finding of pepsin in gastric juice.

Disappointed in his efforts to obtain any new light on the chemistry of the gastric juice, Beaumont enlisted the cooperation of Professor Benjamin Silliman of Yale. Silliman suggested sending some gastric juice to Professor Jons Jacob Berzelius, the famed Swedish chemist, and this was done.

FOURTH SERIES OF EXPERIMENTS, JULY 9 TO NOVEMBER 1, 1833

Filled with great anticipation of Berzelius' investigations, Beaumont and St. Martin went to Plattsburgh to visit his family. He found that his cousin, Dr. Samuel Beaumont, was able to render him material assistance in the work of arranging the data and preparing for the publication of the book. Due to the death of one of his children, Alexis left for Canada, with the promise that he would return to Plattsburgh in the near future. After much military red tape, both Beaumont and St. Martin were stationed in Plattsburgh, where the fourth series of experiments were carried out (Fig. 81). These were done after Beaumont had prepared the manuscript of his previous work for the publisher.

Numbering 62 in all, these experiments were done from July 9 to November 1, 1833. Nothing especially new was brought out in this series, it being largely confirmatory of his previous work.

PUBLICATION OF EXPERIMENTS AND OBSERVATIONS

Beaumont had hoped that additional revelations concerning the chemistry of the gastric juice would be forthcoming from one of his correspondents, but such was not to happen. In December, 1833, one thousand copies of his book were printed. It was entitled "*Experiments and Observations on the Gastric Juice and the Physiology to Digestion,* by William Beaumont, M.D., Surgeon in the United States Army" (Fig. 84). This work, an octavo volume of 280 pages, was printed in Plattsburgh by F. P. Allen, editor of the *Northern Intelligencer* (later the *Northern Sentinel*). The dedication to Joseph Lovell acknowledges in laudatory terms the debts which Beaumont felt he owed his chief (Fig. 85).

Beaumont remarked in the *Preface* of his book: "I submit a body of facts which cannot be invalidated. My opinions may be doubted, denied, or approved, according as they conflict or agree with the opinions of each individual who may read them, but their worth will be best determined by the foundation on which they rest—the incontrovertible facts."

The work is divided into two main portions, the first of which consists of the preliminary observations on the general physiology of digestion and is divided into seven sections:

1. Of Aliment.
2. Of Hunger and Thirst.
3. Of Satisfaction and Satiety.
4. Of Mastication, Insalivation and Deglutition.
5. Of Digestion by the Gastric Juice.
6. Of the Appearance of the Villous Coat, and of the Motions of the Stomach.
7. Of Chylification and Uses of the Bile and Pancreatic Juice.

The greater part of the book is occupied by the detailed account of the 238 experiments and observations (4 series). The work concludes with a series of 51 inferences from the experiments and observations. The second edition of the book was issued from Burlington, Vermont, in 1847, with the same title page, but after "Second Edition" are the words, "Corrected by Samuel Beaumont, M.D." who was Dr. William's cousin.

EXPERIMENTS

AND

OBSERVATIONS

ON THE

GASTRIC JUICE,

AND THE

PHYSIOLOGY OF DIGESTION.

BY WILLIAM BEAUMONT, M. D.

Surgeon in the U. S. Army.

PLATTSBURGH,

PRINTED BY F. P. ALLEN.

1833

Figure 84. Frontispiece of the book which formed the modern foundation of digestive physiology.

TO JOSEPH LOVELL, M. D.

SURGEON GENERAL OF THE UNITED STATES' ARMY,

Whose merit justly entitles him to the rank which he holds,
And whose zeal in the cause of Medical Science is equalled only by his ability to promote it.
As a tribute of respect for his public and private virtues,
And as a feeble acknowledgement for a long tried and unvarying friendship,
This work is respectfully dedicated, by
THE AUTHOR.

Figure 85. William Beaumont's dedication statement to Surgeon-General Lovell, a close personal friend, who enabled him to have a period of detached duty to complete and publish his observations.

LATER LIFE OF BEAUMONT, 1833-53

There being no further occasion for his remaining in Plattsburgh, Beaumont requested and received orders to report to the Surgeon-General in Washington. Sometime prior to this, Beaumont had conceived the idea of asking the Government to remunerate him for the expenses already incurred and to enable him to continue his experiments on digestion, keeping constantly in mind the possibility of taking Alexis abroad for further investigations.

The 23rd Congress was now in session, and before long, Beaumont had succeeded in interesting a number of very prominent men in both houses of Congress. Having received encouragement from practically everyone to whom he applied, Beaumont made his formal petition "memorial" to Congress in the early part of January. He stated that expenses incurred by St. Martin since the injury amounted to not less than $1,000; that the expenses for subsisting, providing for, and retaining St. Martin, money expended and wages paid would amount to $4,000; and that he should be given a stipend of $1.25 per diem for extra duties during the period June 16, 1822 to May 25, 1825, and January 1, 1830 to January 1, 1834, a combined total of $3,148.75. The total amount he requested was $8,148.75. Despite all the appeals, this cause was lost when the motion was defeated by a vote of 129 to 56.

When the 24th Congress convened in the fall of 1835, Beaumont sent another petition to cover his expenses during the experiments. The "memorial" was pigeonholed and has never been heard of from that day to this.

St. Martin had again been permitted to return to his family in Canada, while Beaumont was on an inspection tour in 1834. He promised that he would meet Beaumont in Plattsburgh by June 15 and go with him and his family to the newly assigned post of Jefferson Barracks, 12 miles south of St. Louis (Fig. 78).

St. Martin did not return to Plattsburgh, nor had he sent any message as to his whereabouts or intentions. After considerable delay, Beaumont was forced to leave without him. William Beaumont and Alexis St. Martin never got together again after this.

Beaumont received a letter from St. Martin dated June 26, 1834, while enroute to St. Louis: "DEAR SIR: My wife is not willing for me to go, for she thinks I can do a great deal better to stay at home, for on my farm, she thinks will be a great deal more profit to me. I had started on the 18th of the month and went as far as St. John's and fell sick. On account of that my wife is afraid to let me go . . ."

Jefferson Barracks did not appeal to Beaumont, but he remained there through the summer and fall of 1834. It was about this time that he finally received a reply from Professor Berzelius who said he had not been able to make a satisfactory analysis of the gastric juice.

In November, 1834, Beaumont was granted a three-month leave of absence to return to Plattsburgh and bring his family west, to this, his first permanent post of duty. Such a move, however, proved impractical at the time; and it was not until August, 1835, that Beaumont and family finally settled at the Arsenal, three miles south of St. Louis.

Since there was a second doctor in the barracks, Beaumont felt that he could open an office and give medical attention to citizens as well as soldiers. Within a year, he had built what he termed "a very handsome, lucrative and respectable private practice, with six or eight thousand dollars a year."

Little more than a year after he had moved from the Arsenal to the city, Beaumont was offered the Chair of Surgery in the Medical Department (the first medical department established west of the Mississippi River) which St. Louis University was in the process of establishing. He accepted conditionally, pending approval by the War Department. Unfortunately this plan did not come to fruition. The Medical Department did not open its doors until 1842, and though a course by Beaumont had reached the program stage, there is no evidence that he ever delivered any of the lectures.

During this period, another signal honor was bestowed by Sir Andrew Combe, eminent British physiologist, who reprinted *Experiments and Observations* in Edinburgh, together with a glowing testimonial to Beaumont in its Preface. No doubt, circulation of this reprint greatly enhanced Beaumont's prestige throughout the British Isles and the Continent.

Beaumont had always been of a serious and irascible temperament, and he now had many problems to disturb him. A major change occurred in the War Department that affected seriously his military career: the death, in 1836, of Surgeon-General Lovell and the appointment to that office of Brevet Brigadier General Thomas Lawson. Within a year, word reached Beaumont that he might be transferred back to Jefferson Barracks, and be replaced in St. Louis by Zachary Taylor's son-in-law. Whether or not this was true, it greatly disturbed Beaumont, and he considered the immediate termination of his army service.

On September 18, 1839, General Order No. 48 was issued from the Adjutant General's office in Washington ordering Beaumont to report for duty at Fort Brooks, Florida. Beaumont submitted his resignation, and there followed a long, cumbersome correspondence discussing the circumstances under which a resignation could be honorably submitted and the conditions under which it would be accepted by Washington. This ended on January 20, 1840, with the acceptance of his resignation by order of Major General Macomb, thus drawing to a close Beaumont's brilliant 25-year career as a soldier-surgeon.

Severance of military ties left him free to live and practice as he wished and the years 1840 to his death in 1853 were, for the most part, years of quiet and happiness under almost ideal social and professional conditions. One of the first members of the Medical Society of Missouri, he was elected President of that group in 1840. Twice he entered professional partnerships, but neither worked out and both were soon abandoned.

Only one important challenge to Beaumont's professional skill remained. In the spring of 1849, cholera, carried from New York, swept through St. Louis, finding more than 4,000 victims within four months. Beaumont, then 64 years old, worked day and night through this epidemic, applying every form of treatment and preventative procedure he had found useful many years ago in combatting cholera in the far north.

On a frigid night in March, 1853, when returning home from a professional call, Beaumont slipped and fell, striking his head violently on ice-covered steps. Soon afterwards he developed a carbuncle on his neck, complicated by a severe fever, and on April 25, 1853, William Beaumont died.

His wife, Deborah, lived until January 23, 1870. They were buried side by side in Bellefontaine Cemetery, St. Louis, their graves marked by simple markers. Members of the St. Louis University School of Medicine make a pilgrimage to the cemetery on the anniversary of his death.

LATER LIFE OF ST. MARTIN, 1834-1880

Beaumont failed repeatedly to get in touch with St. Martin after his transfer to St. Louis, though he clung for many years to the faint hope that he might some day resume his tests with St. Martin. He kept alive every contact, especially through Mr. Morrison of the American Fur Company, and he corresponded directly with St. Martin after the latter had been located in Canada. Beaumont's heirs, in fact, found among his papers at least 60 letters on the subject.

St. Martin himself blew alternately hot and cold in dealing with proposals to return. In one respect, however, all reports agreed: the man was a born spendthrift and regardless of his immediate fortunes, his chronic condition was one of abject poverty.

St. Martin lived 28 years after the death of Beaumont. Nothing further was accomplished in the nature of experiments except some tests by Francis Gurney Smith, professor of the Institute of Medicine in the Medical Department of Pennsylvania College, with the aid of Professor R. E. Rodgers (*Medical Examiner,* July, 1856). It seems that St. Martin was exhibiting himself at different medical schools in the East and was also reported at Buffalo about this time. In 1879, he returned to St. Thomas de Joliette in Canada, where he passed his last days in poverty. St. Martin knew none of the comfort and happiness that Beaumont enjoyed.

Even his death on June 24, 1880, did not end the controversy his accident had created. St. Martin's family had refused all requests for an autopsy, including an offer of a fair price by the eminent Sir William Osler, then a resident at McGill Institute in Montreal. On the day of St. Martin's death, Osler had received the following telegram: "Don't come for autopsy, will be killed." In accordance with the family's wishes, St. Martin's body was buried in the cemetery of St. Thomas de Jolietta Parish, Quebec, in an unmarked grave dug 8 feet below the surface to prevent exhumation. The body had also been kept home much longer than usual and during a hot spell of weather so as to allow decomposition to set in.

Not until July, 1960, was this grave located by a committee of the Canadian Federation of Biological Societies, with the aid of an 86-year-old granddaughter of St. Martin.

Half a century ago, the great Lord Berkely Moynihan[4] wrote: "As we look backward upon the long history of the science and art of medicine, we seem to see a great procession of famous and heroic figures. . . . They now belong not to one country but to every country, for they are the common possession and the pride of all the world. . . . They are men whose deeds will not be forgotten, and whose names will live to all generations."

Such a name is William Beaumont, who left a legacy to the medical profession of greater magnitude than is generally realized (Fig. 86). There is no argument that his experiments on Alexis St. Martin established the basic principles of digestion. The role of hydrochloric acid was established and many of the principles of human digestion have persisted to this day. As Dragstedt pointed out in his address before the American College of Surgeons in 1970, he was the first surgical scientist in the United States. His experiments stimulated physiologic research on human digestion which gradually spread throughout the world.

The careful and detailed postoperative progress notes made on his famous patient were quite informative and complete. He might well be designated as the "Godfather of the Ideal Progress Note!" If every physician was as thorough as Beaumont in recording postoperative and progress notes, the problem of malpractice would be greatly reduced.

Another legacy of Beaumont was his courage in asking and gaining permission to treat civilians as well as military patients. If he had not received official permission to "moonlight" while assigned to Mackinac Island, it probably would have made it impossible for him to attend Alexis St. Martin, which led to his historic physiologic observations.

Another legacy was foresight in seeking the help of basic scientists in helping solve his problem. His collaborative study

BEAUMONT INFERENCES
EFFECTS ON DIGESTION AND STOMACH

Aids: **Animal over vegetable**
Minuteness and tenderness
Bulk and nutriment necessary

Hinders: **Oily foods**
Excess quantity
Condiments

Ardent spirits produce diseases of stomach

Figure 86. The experiments of Dr. William Beaumont developed the early foundation of clinical dietetics.

with Professor Dunglison made possible the identification of muriatic or hydrochloric acid. Professor Silliman of the Chemistry Department of Yale University also contributed to the identification of the acid involved in human digestion. In recent years, the principle of combining basic science "know-how" in clinical practice as introduced by Beaumont has been widely adopted.

The principle of reconfirming data before publication was widely practiced by Beaumont. This enabled him to be absolutely certain of his observations, although it meant a delay in the publication of his monumental observations. The principle of "publish or perish" was not as well established as in the twentieth century, or he might have published a hundred papers based on his 238 experiments.

In these days when the majority of physicians have had military duty, they might well recall the assistance provided by the Army to insure the contributions of Beaumont, despite primitive conditions. For example, Surgeon General Lovell, the first surgeon-general of the army, made it possible for Beaumont to be on detached duty to repeat and reconfirm his observations. The army also made the Canadian citizen a sergeant in the American Army in order to lighten the financial burden of his maintenance from the shoulders of Beaumont. General Lovell also supported the request of $10,000 from Congress to recompense Beaumont for providing maintainance of Alexis St. Martin for several years. This request, as well as a second one, was not favorably acted upon by Congress.

Finally, it might be recalled that great contributions by Beaumont were made without a prolonged college education and only two years of preceptorship training in medicine. He was trained by his preceptor to make frequent and accurate observations which were meticulously recorded. This training served to make Beaumont a compulsive diarist. His background might well be used to support the current trend toward a shortened curriculum.

Dr. John F. Fulton, in the foreward to Rosen's *The Reception of William Beaumont's Discoveries in Europe,* wrote[6]: "William Beaumont may be ranked with Benjamin Franklin and Weir Mitchell as one of the three Americans whose writings have exerted a profound influence upon medical thought of Europe prior to 1900. . . . On the basis of one well studied case, Beaumont was able to change the course of medical thought in the sphere of gastroenterology."

REFERENCES

1. Beaumont, W.: *Experiments and Observations on the Gastric Juice and the Physiology of Digestions.* Plattsburg, printed by F. P. Allen, 1933.
2. Beaumont, W.: *Little Journeys to the Homes of Great Physicians.* St. Louis, Mosby, 4-28, 1937.
3. Cushing, H.: William Beaumont's Rendezvous with Fame. *Yale J Biol Med,* 8:113, 1935.
4. Franklin, A. W. (Ed.): *Selected Writings of Lord Moynihan.* (A Centenary Volume For the Osler Club of London). London, Pitman Medical Publishing, 1967.
5. Meyer, J. S.: *Life and Letters of Dr. William Beaumont.* St. Louis, Mosby, 1939.
6. Rosen, G.: *The Reception of William Beaumont's Discovery in Europe.* New York, Schuman's, 1942.
7. Selleck, H. B.: *Beaumont and The Mackinac Island Miracle.* East Lansing, Beaumont Memorial Foundation, 1971.

Name Index

C

H

I

L

M

N

O

P

Q

R

W

Y

Z

Subject Index